Atlas of Gynecologic Cytology

Grace T McKee
Formerly Associate Pathologist, Massachusetts General Hospital, and
Associate Professor, Harvard Medical School, Boston

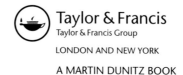

Taylor & Francis
Taylor & Francis Group

LONDON AND NEW YORK

A MARTIN DUNITZ BOOK

First published in the United Kingdom in 2004 by
Taylor & Francis, an imprint of the Taylor & Francis Group,
2 Park Square, Milton Park, Abingdon, Oxfordshire, OX14 4RN.

Tel.:	+44 (0) 20 7583 9855
Fax.:	+44 (0) 20 7842 2298
E-mail:	info@dunitz.co.uk
Website:	http://www.dunitz.co.uk

A CIP record for this book is available from the British Library.

Library of Congress Cataloging-in-Publication Data

Data available on application

ISBN 1 84184 411 X

Distributed in North and South America by
Taylor & Francis
2000 NW Corporate Blvd
Boca Raton, FL 33431, USA

Within Continental USA
Tel: 800 272 7737; Fax: 800 374 3401
Outside Continental USA
Tel: 561 994 0555; Fax: 561 361 6018
E-mail   orders@crcpress.com

Distributed in the rest of the world by
Thomson Publishing Services
Cheriton House
North Way
Andover, Hampshire SP10 5BE, UK
Tel.:   +44 (0)1264 332424
E-mail: salesorder.tandf@thomsonpublishingservices.co.uk

Production editor: Julian Evans
Composition by EXPO Holdings, Malaysia
Printed and bound in Spain by Grafos SA

Contents

1 The normal Pap smear

The routine Papanicolaou (Pap) smear (cervical smear) is a well-accepted screening test that has been demonstrated to lower the mortality rate from carcinoma of the cervix. Traditionally, the Pap smear was prepared by spreading material obtained from the exo- and endocervix on a glass slide. With this method, most of the material is discarded, being impossible to remove from the spatula or brush. Thus, although the conventional Pap smear may contain 300–500 000 cells, it may not contain representative cells from a lesion present on the cervix. It is impossible to spread the material evenly when it is done manually, resulting in thick areas and very thinly spread, air-dried areas. Another often encountered problem is the location of abnormal cells at the edge of the slide, sometimes just outside the coverslip. With liquid-based cytological preparations, on the other hand, almost all of the material removed from the cervix is in the vial and therefore lesional cells are invariably present on the slide. The cellular material is evenly spread on the slide and abnormal cells are scattered throughout the smear. The area containing cells is a larger circle in ThinPrep® smears, measuring 20 mm and 13 mm in SurePath® preparations. As both liquid-based preparations contain approximately 70 000 cells, it is not surprising that in SurePath® smears many of the cells lie above other cells in different planes of focus. Cell clusters appear darker in SurePath® than in ThinPrep® preparations. Liquid-based preparations are much easier to screen than conventional smears and do not contain the usual artifacts of endocervical cells tucked under mucin, obscuring blood and polymorphs, or air-drying and 'cornflakes'. They are also superior to conventional smears for detection of abnormalities. ThinPrep® picks up a higher number of low grade squamous intraepithelial lesion (LSIL) and high grade squamous intraepithelial lesion (HSIL) cases compared with conventional smears; SurePath® picks up a higher number of LSIL cases and an equal number of HSIL cases.

For a liquid-based preparation to be adequate there should be at least 5000 well-visualized squamous cells in the smear. For ThinPrep®, this equates to 50 cells per 10× field. The absence of endocervical or metaplastic cells does not render the smear inadequate or suboptimal. Their presence denotes sampling of the squamocolumnar junction, where most dysplasias are believed to arise. With conventional smears, the best time for smear-taking is mid cycle as this precludes unsatisfactory results due to extensive cytolysis (luteal or secretory phase) or obscuring blood (menstrual smear). Blood is not an issue with liquid-based cytology as red blood cells are lysed in ThinPrep® and SurePath® processing. Excessive neutrophil polymorphs often obscure cellular detail with conventional smears. With ThinPrep®, the polymorphs tend to form small clumps or may be seen singly in the background, not obscuring the squamous cells. Similarly, the epithelial cells

Table 1.1
Comparison of ThinPrep®, SurePath®, and conventional smears

ThinPrep®	SurePath®	Conventional smear
All material in vial	All material in vial	Most material discarded
Virtual monolayer	Even, but thick layer	Unevenly spread
Cells within circle	Cells in and outside circle	Material all over slide
70 000 cells approximately including lesional cells	70 000 cells approximately including lesional cells	300–500 000 cells approximately. Lesional cells may be absent
RBCs lysed	RBCs not present	RBCs obscure when present
WBCs present	WBCs usually not present	WBCs usually obscure
Clusters translucent	Clusters thick and dark	Thick and thinner areas
ECs single, small groups	ECs in large clumps that are often 'feathered'	ECs often smeared in mucin
Single ECs columnar	Single ECs columnar but may flatten like histiocytes	Single ECs columnar
EMs small, also single	EMs appear larger with abundant cytoplasm	EMs in large clusters with abundant histiocytes
Dysplastic nuclei may be dark or pale	Dysplastic nuclei may be dark or pale	Dysplastic nuclei may be dark or pale
Tumor diathesis clumps	Tumor diathesis clumps	Tumor diathesis smeared all over slide

RBCs, red blood cells; WBCs, white blood cells; ECs, endocervical cells; EMs, endometrial cells

are not obscured by polymorphs with SurePath® as the gradient containing polymorphs is discarded when the smear is being prepared. If neutrophils are seen in a SurePath® smear it is a sign of inflammation. Mucin is often seen in abundance in conventional smears, but in much smaller amounts in liquid-based preparations. (See Table 1.1.)

The normal constituents of a Pap smear comprise squamous and glandular epithelial cells, histiocytes, neutrophil polymorphs, some blood, and mucin. Occasionally other structures may be seen, such as psammoma bodies and contaminants in the form of pollen grains or alternaria. A Pap smear can usually provide information relating to the hormonal status of a woman, whether she is pre- or postmenopausal, and the phase of the menstrual cycle. The fallacy with well-estrogenized smears is that many postmenopausal women are on hormone replacement

therapy, and therefore have a mature smear pattern, often with endometrial cells. Thus, clinical information is vital for accurate interpretation.

In the absence of information about an intrauterine device (IUD), a smear with atypical endometrial cells may be misdiagnosed as indicative of adenocarcinoma. In similar vein, it is useful for the cytopathologist/cytotechnologist to know that a patient has had chemo- or radiation therapy as both can lead to abnormal cells in the Pap smear. In addition to detecting abnormal cells that might develop into neoplasia and other malignant lesions of the cervix or vagina, including metastatic tumors, Pap smears are useful for detecting more mundane changes, such as infections. Various devices are used for procuring material from the cervix, some sampling both the endocervix and ectocervix, others just one or the other.

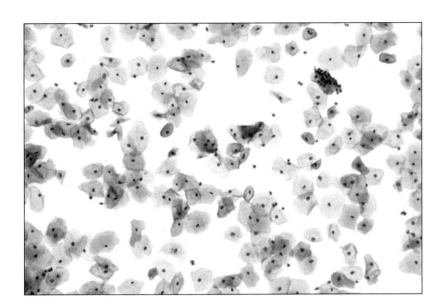

Figure 1.1

Normal smear pattern, mid cycle

This field shows a mature smear pattern composed of superficial and intermediate cells with a clean background. Note that polymorphs form a small clump in the top right corner and do not obscure the epithelial cells in ThinPrep®. (Pap LP ThinPrep®)

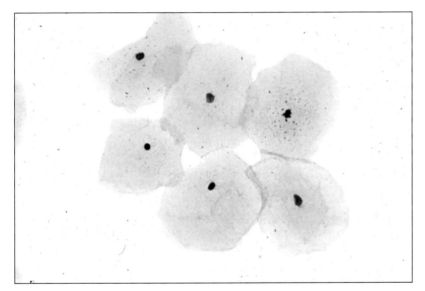

Figure 1.2

Superficial cells

These superficial cells have a polygonal shape and pyknotic nuclei. Note that superficial cells can be cyanophilic as well as acidophilic. The presence of superficial cells is indicative of high levels of circulating estrogen. (Pap LP ThinPrep®)

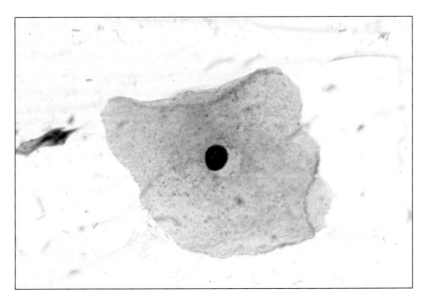

Figure 1.3

Superficial cells

Superficial cells are large and polygonal with translucent acidophilic (pink) cytoplasm and pyknotic nuclei. (Pap OI Conventional smear)

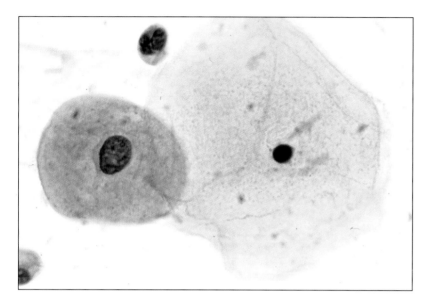

Figure 1.4

Superficial and parabasal cells

The superficial cell is much larger than the parabasal cell in this field. The parabasal cell is clearly visible although partially covered by the superficial cell due to the translucency of the cytoplasm of the latter. (Pap OI Conventional smear)

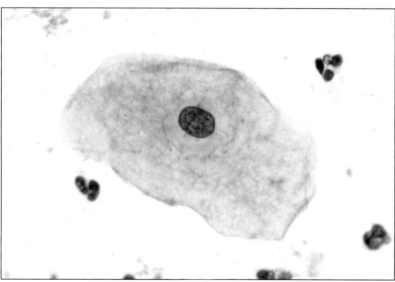

Figure 1.5

Intermediate cell

This is a large polygonal cell with a vesicular nucleus that is roughly the size of a polymorph (and of an endometrial cell), with translucent cytoplasm that is not as dense as that of squamous metaplastic cells. The cytoplasm usually stains blue. (Pap OI ThinPrep®: intermed cells)

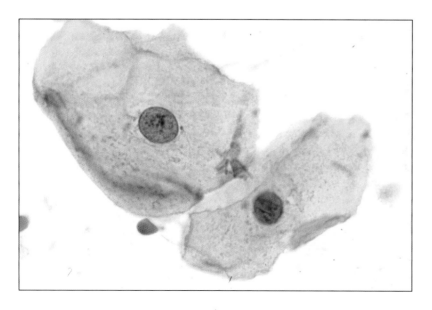

Figure 1.6

Intermediate cells

These two intermediate cells exhibit folded edges. This folding of the cytoplasmic edges is usually seen in smears taken at mid cycle. (Pap OI Conventional smear)

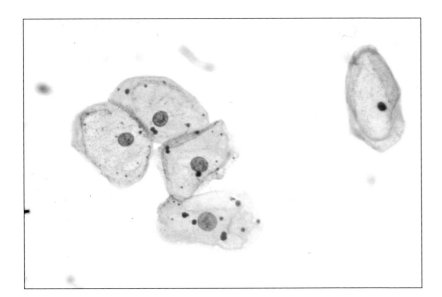

Figure 1.7

Keratohyaline granules

The intermediate cells in this field contain variably sized keratohyaline granules. (Pap HP Conventional smear)

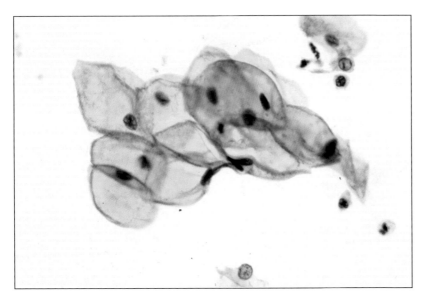

Figure 1.8

Navicular cells

A ThinPrep® smear showing a sheet of navicular cells with eccentric nuclei and thickened edges. These should not be mistaken for koilocytes. The clear cytoplasm contains glycogen and does not represent a halo. (Pap HP ThinPrep®)

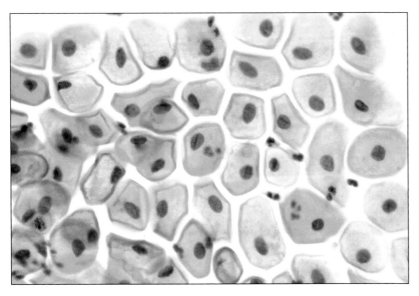

Figure 1.9

Navicular cells

A SurePath® smear showing navicular cells in a mosaic-type arrangement. Note the thickened cytoplasmic rims and glycogen, though not all the cells have eccentric nuclei. (Pap HP SurePath®)

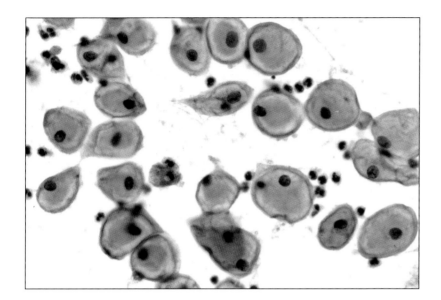

Figure 1.10

Navicular cells

These cells are traditionally described as boat-shaped and are more commonly seen in smears taken during pregnancy. (Pap HP Conventional smear)

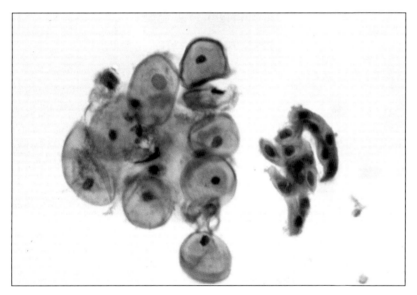

Figure 1.11

Parabasal cells

There are two groups of parabasal cells in this field. The cells in the group on the left are more mature as they are larger and have more cytoplasm than the more immature cells in the group on the right. (Pap HP ThinPrep®)

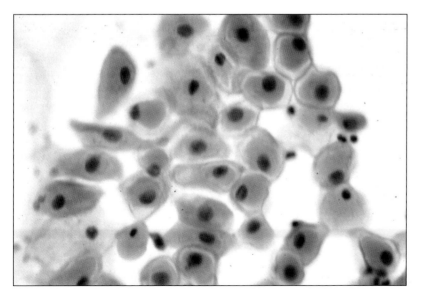

Figure 1.12

Parabasal cells

This vaginal smear shows parabasal cells with a high nuclear : cytoplasmic ratio and a thickened cytoplasmic edge, containing glycogen, resembling navicular cells. (Pap HP SurePath®)

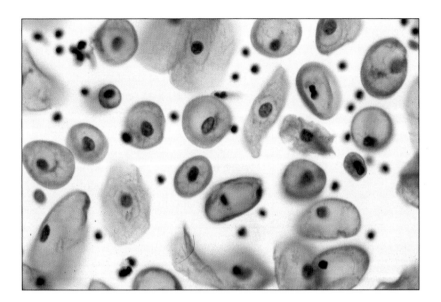

Figure 1.13

Parabasal cells

Single parabasal cells are seen in this postmenopausal smear, some with a thickened cytoplasmic rim. A similar pattern is often seen in postpartum smears. (Pap HP SurePath®)

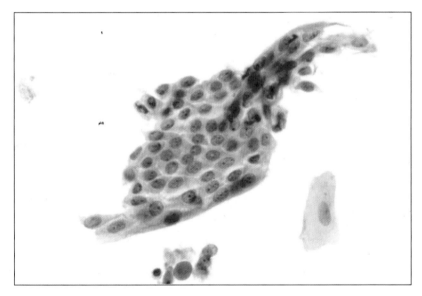

Figure 1.14

Parabasal cells

This sheet of parabasal cells shows uniform nuclei but a high nuclear : cytoplasmic ratio. Small nucleoli are present. Parabasal cells are often seen in sheets in atrophic smears. If there is doubt as to whether these cells are atypical, a 5-day course of topical estrogen may be recommended to mature the cervical epithelium and a repeat smear taken to detect any abnormalities present. (Pap LP ThinPrep®)

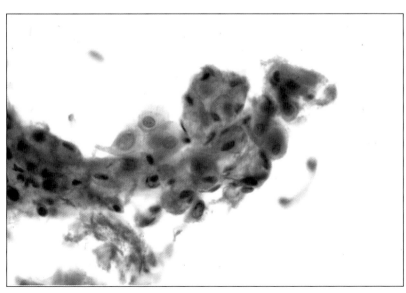

Figure 1.15

Parabasal cells

Parabasal cells with a high nuclear : cytoplasmic ratio are interspersed with endocervical cells containing pale pink mucin in this atrophic smear. The two types of cells are easily distinguishable in ThinPrep smears but often are more difficult to separate in some conventional smears. (Pap HP ThinPrep®)

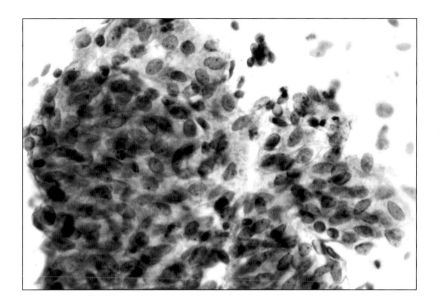

Figure 1.16

Parabasal cells

This large group of parabasal cells contains nuclei that range from ovoid to spindle-shaped. Occasionally, only spindle-shaped parabasal cells are seen in the smear, especially in women who have been menopausal for decades. In well-fixed smears grooves are often seen in parabasal cells. (Pap HP Conventional smear)

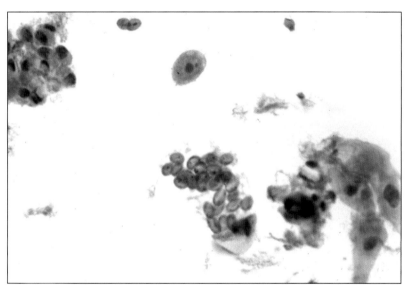

Figure 1.17

Parabasal cells

Intermediate and parabasal cells are seen, with a clump of small bare nuclei. These represent stripped parabasal cell nuclei, not endometrial cells. Bare nuclei are often seen in atrophic smears, in large numbers in conventional smears, and fewer in liquid-based preparations. (Pap HP ThinPrep®)

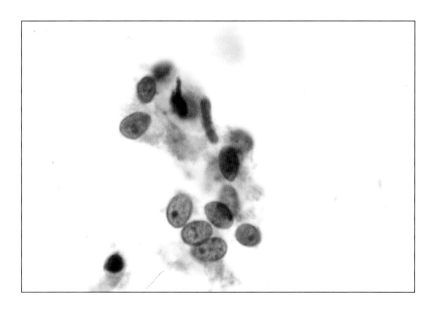

Figure 1.18

Parabasal cells

Bare parabasal cell nuclei are seen in this field, some ovoid with small nucleoli, others more spindled. (Pap OI ThinPrep®)

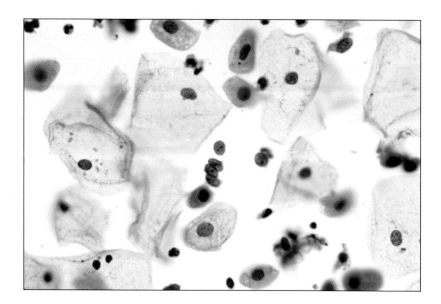

Figure 1.19

Parabasal cells

Note the small group of bare parabasal cell nuclei in the center of this field, surrounded by parabasal and intermediate cells. (Pap HP SurePath®)

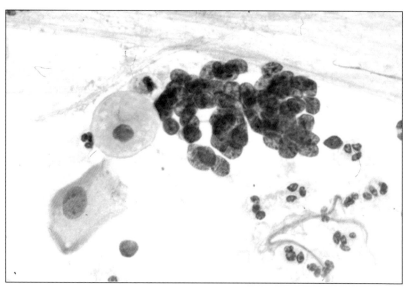

Figure 1.20

Parabasal cells

This field shows a collection of bare parabasal cell nuclei with two intact parabasal cells. Note the air-dried polymorphs in this conventional smear. (Pap HP Conventional smear)

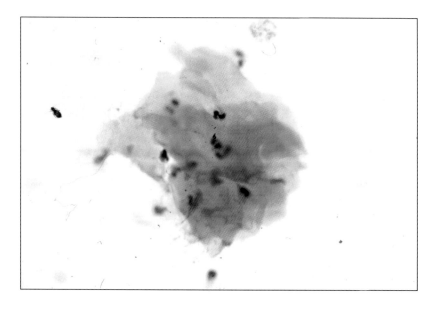

Figure 1.21

Anucleate squamous cells

This cluster of keratinized anucleated squamous cells is indicative of hyperkeratosis. Keratin is not normally seen in the cervix and its presence signifies some irritant, such as a ring pessary, or it may indicate vulval contaminant. (Pap LP ThinPrep®)

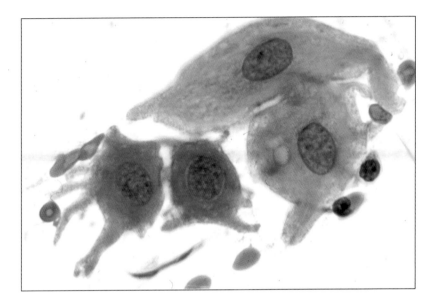

Figure 1.22

Squamous metaplasia

Small immature squamous metaplastic cells are seen on the left with large, more mature metaplastic cells on the right that are approaching parabasal cell size. (Pap HP Conventional smear)

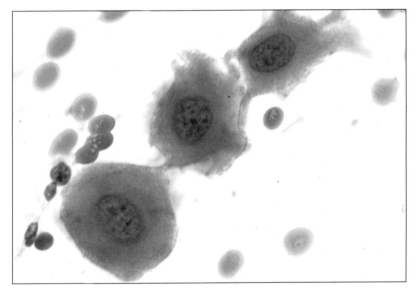

Figure 1.23

Squamous metaplasia

Squamous metaplastic cells display dense blue cytoplasm, darker than that of intermediate cells, and not as translucent. Note the 'pulled-out' cytoplasm of the cells, a feature more commonly observed in conventional smears than in liquid-based preparations (personal observation). (Pap HP Conventional smear)

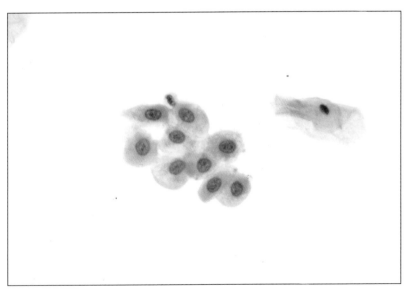

Figure 1.24

Squamous metaplasia

A sheet of squamous metaplastic cells with a high nuclear/cytoplasmic ratio. Note their small size compared with the blue-staining superficial cell with its pyknotic nucleus. (Pap HP ThinPrep®)

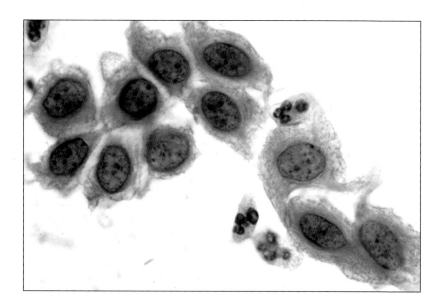

Figure 1.25

Immature squamous metaplasia

Conventional smear showing immature squamous metaplastic cells with typical 'pulled-out' cytoplasm, high nuclear : cytoplasmic ratio and hyperchromatic nuclei. These are small cells using the polymorphs as a size gauge. (Pap HP Conventional smear)

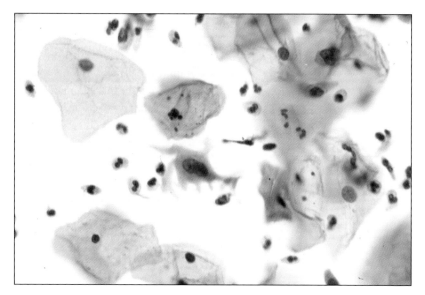

Figure 1.26

Immature squamous metaplasia

In the center of the field is a small binucleate metaplastic cell, surrounded by superficial and intermediate cells and neutrophil polymorphs. (Pap HP SurePath®)

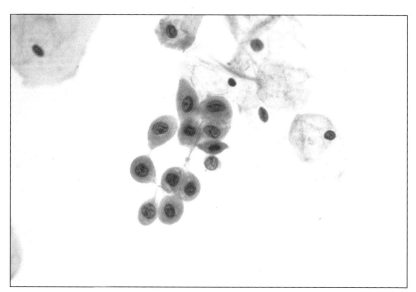

Figure 1.27

Immature squamous metaplasia

These small cells with sharply defined cytoplasmic borders, dense cytoplasm (compared with that of the adjacent intermediate cells), and a high nuclear : cytoplasmic ratio are immature squamous metaplastic cells. Note the nuclear grooves. (Pap HP ThinPrep®)

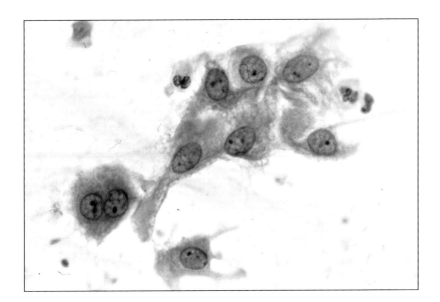

Figure 1.28

Immature squamous metaplasia

Conventional smear showing so-called 'spider cells' with exaggeration of the 'pulled-out' cytoplasm. Note the high nuclear : cytoplasmic ratio, round nuclei and nucleoli, the latter indicative of reactive changes. (Pap HP Conventional smear)

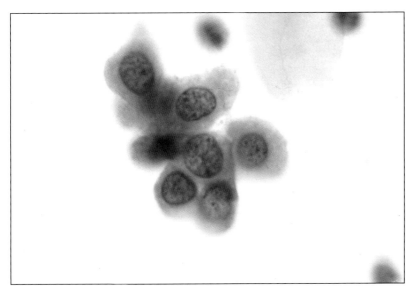

Figure 1.29

Immature squamous metaplasia

Small metaplastic cells are seen here, with dense cytoplasm (note that high grade dysplastic cells can have dense or delicate cytoplasm), round nuclei and coarse but evenly distributed chromatin. (Pap HP ThinPrep®)

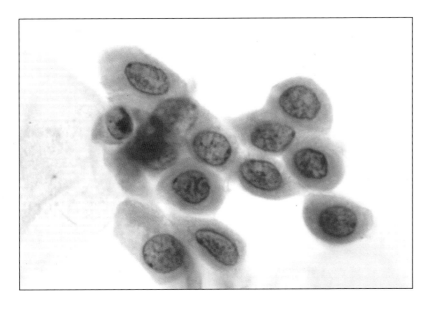

Figure 1.30

Immature squamous metaplasia

These small cells show metaplastic features, namely dense cytoplasm, high nuclear : cytoplasmic ratio, and formation of a flat sheet. Although there is slight nuclear irregularity these are not high grade dysplastic cells. (Pap HP ThinPrep®)

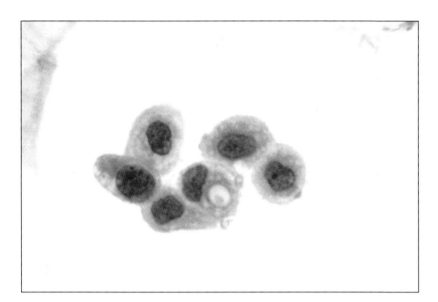

Figure 1.31

Immature squamous metaplasia

These cells have a high nuclear : cytoplasmic ratio, may have small nucleoli and often show degenerative vacuoles within their dense cytoplasm, as illustrated here. The crinkly nuclear margin irregularities are also indicative of degenerative changes. (Pap HP ThinPrep®)

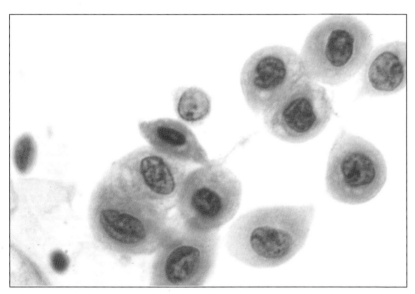

Figure 1.32

Immature squamous metaplasia

These metaplastic cells are slightly larger with more cytoplasm than those in the previous images. In some cells the dense cytoplasm is pulled out in typical metaplastic cell fashion; also there is some nuclear irregularity. (Pap HP ThinPrep®)

Recommended reading

1. Klinkhammer PJ, Meerding WJ, Rosier PF, Hanselaar AG. Liquid-based cervical cytology. *Cancer* 2003;**99**:263–71.

2. Negri G, Menia E, Egarter-Vig E, et al. ThinPrep versus conventional Papanicolaou smear in the cytologic follow-up of women with equivocal cervical smears. *Cancer* 2003;**99**:342–5.

3. Ugar DS, Eltabbakh GH, Mount SL. Positive predictive value of liquid-based and conventional cervical Papanicolaou smears reported as malignant. *Gynecol Oncol* 2003;**89**:227–32.

4. Abulafia O, Pezzullo JC, Sherer DM. Performance of ThinPrep liquid-based cervical cytology in comparison with conventionally prepared Papanicolaou smears: quantitative survey. *Gynecol Oncol* 2003;**90**:137–44.

5. Cheung AN, Szeto ER, Leung BS, et al. Liquid-based cytology and conventional cervical smears: a comparison study in an Asian screening population. *Cancer* 2003;**99**:331–5.

6. Monsonego J, Autillo-Touati A, Bergeron C, et al. Liquid-based cytology for primary cervical cancer screening: a multi-centre study. *Br J Cancer* 2001;**84**:360–6.

7. Ferris DG, Heidemann NL, Litaker MS, et al. The efficacy of liquid-based cervical cytology using direct-to-vial sample collection. *J Fam Pract* 2000;**49**:1005–11.

8. Chhieng DC, Talley LI, Roberson J, et al. Intgerovserver variability: comparison between liquid-based and conventional preparations in gynecologic cytology. *Cancer* 2002;**96**:67–73.

9. Baker JJ. Conventional and liquid-based cervicovaginal cytology: a comparison study with clinical and histologic follow-up. *Diagn Cytopathol* 2002;**27**:185–8.

10. Sass MA. Use of a liquid-based, thin-layer Pap test in a community hospital: Impact on cytology performance and productivity. *Acta Cytol* 2004;**48**:17–22.

11. Studeman KD, Ioffe OB, Puszkiewicz J, et al. Effect of cellularity on the sensitivity of detecting squamous lesions in liquid-based cervical cytology. *Acta Cytol* 2003;**47**:605–10.

12. Linder J, Zahniser DS. The ThinPrep Pap test. A review of clinical studies. *Acta Cytol* 1997;**41**:30–8.

13. Williamson BA, De Frias D, Gunn R, et al. Significance of extensive hyperkeratosis on cervical/vaginal smears. *Acta Cytol* 2003;**47**:749–52.

14. Malle D, Pateinakis P, Chakka E, Destouni C. Experience with a thin-layer, liquid-based cervical cytologic screening method. *Acta Cytol* 2003;**47**:129–34.

15. Biscotti CV, O'Brien DL, Gero MA, et al. Thin-layer Pap test vs. conventional Pap smear. Analysis of 400 split samples. *J Reprod Med* 2002;**47**:9–13.

16. Bolick DR, Hellman DJ. Laboratroy implementation and efficacy assessment of the ThinPrep cervical cancer screening system. *Acta Cytol* 1998;**42**:209–13.

17. Marino JF, Fremont-Smith M. Direct-to-vial experience with AutoCytePREP in a small New England regional cytology practice. *J Reprod Med* 2001;**46**:353–8.

18. Davey DD. Cervical cytology classification and the Bethesda system. *Cancer* 2003;**9**:327–34.

2 Normal glandular constituents

The presence of endocervical and/or squamous metaplastic cells is no longer required for a Pap smear to be adequate according to the new Bethesda guidelines. These cells indicate that the squamocolumnar junction has been sampled, provided at least 10 cells are present in liquid-based preparations. Both these types of cells may be in sheets or small groups, or single. Endocervical cells appear to be more numerous in SurePath® samples and are often single in ThinPreps®. They vary in shape in normal smears, as seen in the accompanying figures.

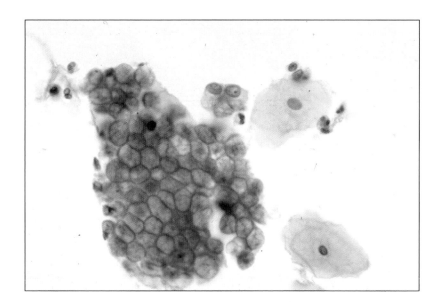

Figure 2.1

Endocervical cells

This is a small sheet of endocervical cells displaying honeycombing. The cytoplasm of endocervical cells is delicate and foamy and the nuclei in focus adjacent to the upper squamous cell at 2 o'clock are slightly bigger than the neutrophils in the field. (Pap HP ThinPrep®)

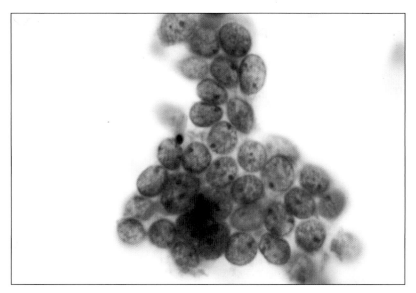

Figure 2.2

Endocervical cells

A sheet of endocervical cells showing uniformity, round nuclei, and vesicular chromatin. (Pap OI ThinPrep®)

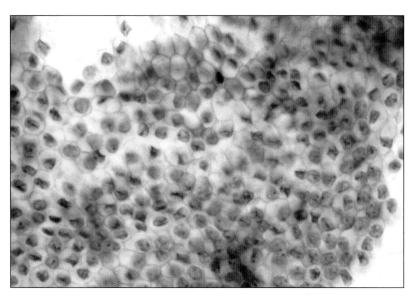

Figure 2.3

Endocervical cells

In conventional smears, endocervical cells are often seen in large sheets, sometimes entangled in mucin, and often in the form of stripped or bare nuclei. Stripped endocervical nuclei are rare in ThinPrep® smears. This is a large sheet of endocervical cells with clearly defined honeycombing of the cytoplasm. (Pap HP Conventional smear)

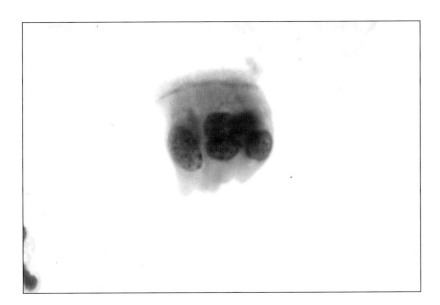

Figure 2.4

Endocervical cells

These three endocervical cells have clearly visible pink-staining cilia. Ciliated endocervicals may be seen in normal smears and should not be assumed to suggest tubal metaplasia without other corroborating evidence. (Pap OI ThinPrep®)

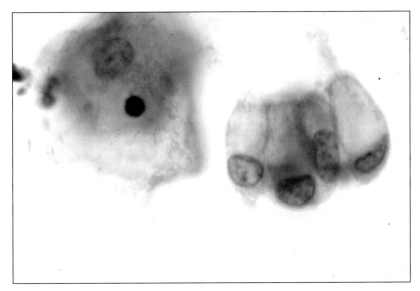

Figure 2.5

Endocervical cells

The tall columnar shape of endocervical cells is clearly seen here. Note that the mucin within the cytoplasm compresses the nucleus in the cell on the right. (Pap LP ThinPrep®)

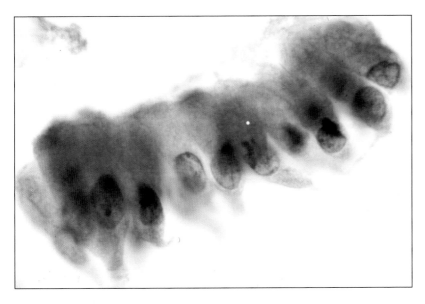

Figure 2.6

Endocervical cells

These tall columnar endocervical cells are forming a picket fence arrangement. (Pap OI ThinPrep®)

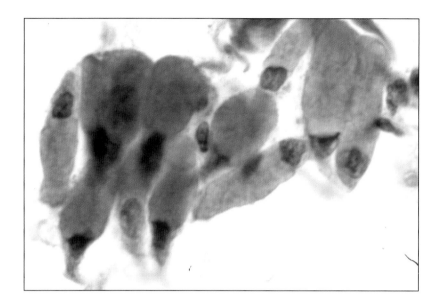

Figure 2.7

Endocervical cells

The endocervical cells shown here are distended with mucin, which in some cells causes flattening of the nucleus. (Pap OI ThinPrep®)

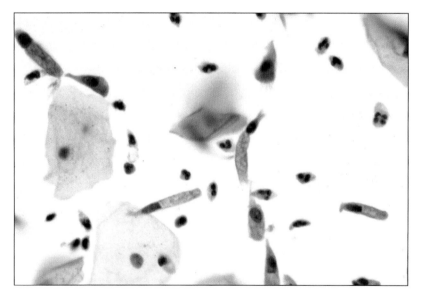

Figure 2.8

Endocervical cells

Although endocervical cells are usually seen in thick clusters in SurePath® slides, single tall columnar endocervical cells are not uncommon. (Pap HP SurePath®)

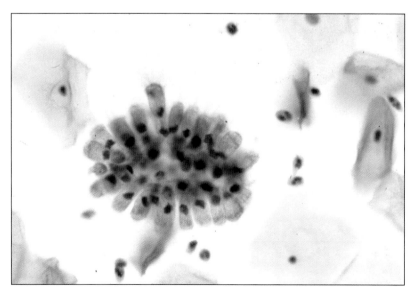

Figure 2.9

Endocervical cells

This rosette is not indicative of adenocarcinoma *in situ*. The nuclei at the base of the cells are at the center of the rosette. This appearance is not uncommon in SurePath® smears but is also seen in endocervical brush samples prepared as conventional smears. (Pap HP SurePath®)

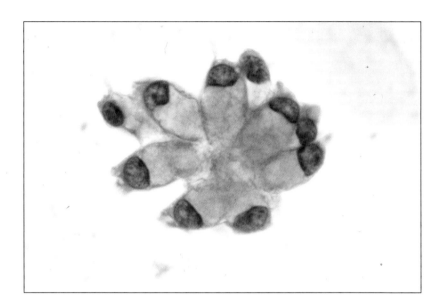

Figure 2.10

Endocervical cells

Another example of a benign rosette, this one in a ThinPrep® smear. (Pap OI ThinPrep®)

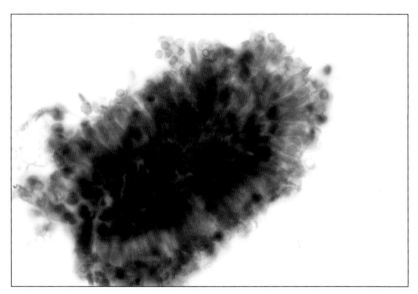

Figure 2.11

Endocervical cells

In this SurePath® preparation, tall columnar endocervical cells form a tight cluster entrapping intact red blood cells. (Pap HP SurePath®)

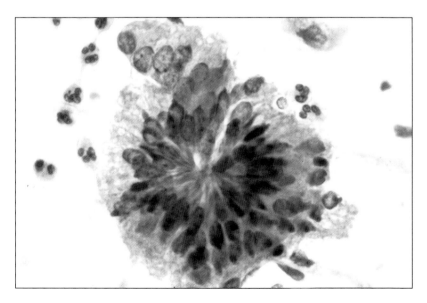

Figure 2.12

Endocervical cells

Endocervical cells are forming a pseudorosette with the base of the cells towards the center, in this conventional endocervical brush smear. (Pap HP Conventional smear)

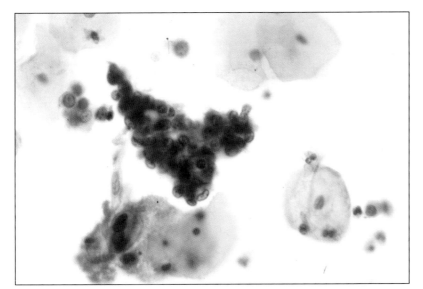

Figure 2.13

Endometrial cells

In the center of the field is a cluster of crowded, small glandular cells, some with irregular nuclei. Not much cytoplasm is present compared with the abundant cytoplasm seen in SurePath® preparations (see Figure 2.20). Endometrial cells may be seen from the first to day 10 of the menstrual cycle, although some authorities allow their appearance up to day 12. The cluster bears some resemblance to a mulberry. (Pap HP ThinPrep®)

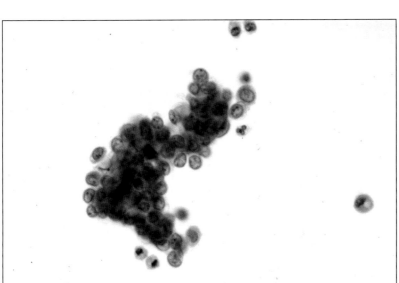

Figure 2.14

Endometrial cells

A tight cluster of small endometrial cells with minimal cytoplasm, vesicular nuclei with clearly visible chromatin detail and variable nuclear size and shape. (Pap HP ThinPrep®)

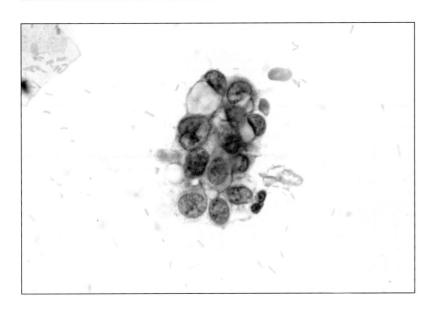

Figure 2.15

Endometrial cells

A cluster of endometrial cells showing nuclei varying from round to somewhat irregular, and vacuolated cytoplasm. (Pap HP Conventional smear)

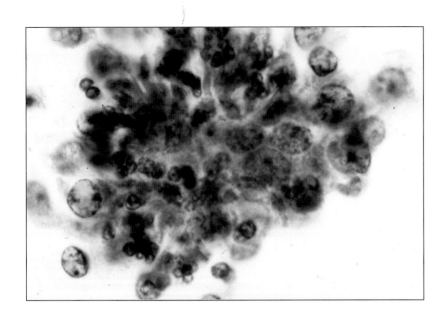

Figure 2.16

Endometrial cells, hematoidin crystals

A cluster of endometrial cells. Note that the nuclei are slightly larger than the lymphocytes and neutrophils within the cluster. Note the reddish-orange hematoidin crystals. (Pap HP ThinPrep®)

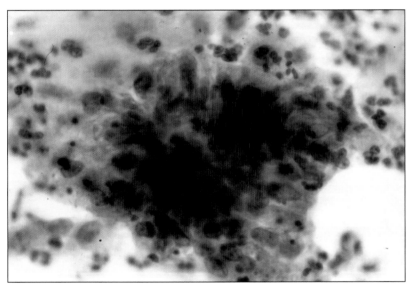

Figure 2.17

Hematoidin crystals

Orange crystals in rosette formation overlie and obscure the endometrial cells and neutrophils in this field. (Pap OI Conventional smear)

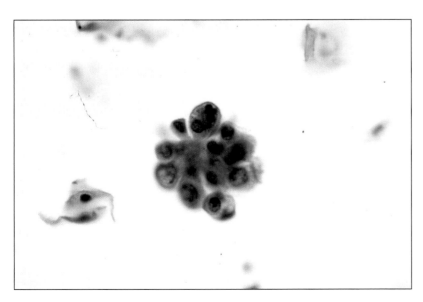

Figure 2.18

Endometrial cells

A three-dimensional cluster of small glandular cells with varying amounts of cytoplasm is noted in this field. In this preparation, cells lie in several different planes on the smear, thus the background cells appear out of focus. (Pap LP SurePath®)

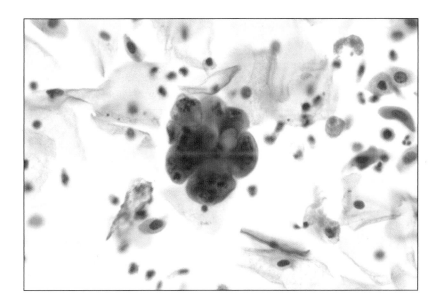

Figure 2.19

Endometrial cells

Note the cluster of endometrial cells showing vacuolation and prominent nucleoli. These appearances are within normal limits for endometrial cells in SurePath® smears. (Pap HP SurePath®)

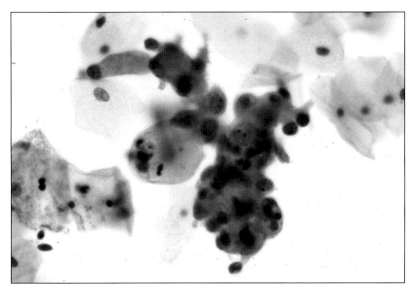

Figure 2.20

Endometrial cells

Clusters of endometrial cells with abundant cytoplasm are seen here. Note the contrasting tall columnar endocervical cell at 11 o'clock for comparison. (Pap HP SurePath®)

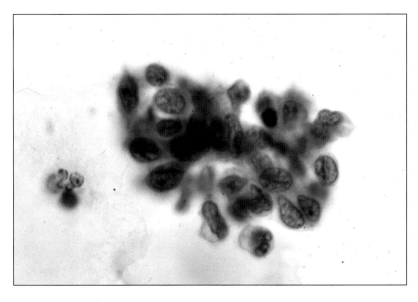

Figure 2.21

Endometrial stromal cells

A cluster of endometrial cells with admixed spindle-shaped stromal cells. Note the polymorph at 9 o'clock for size comparison. (Pap HP ThinPrep®)

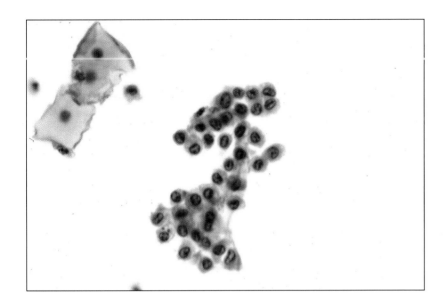

Figure 2.22

Endometrial histiocytes

A collection of small histiocytic cells, referred to as 'endometrial histiocytes' by some authorities, and as 'endometrial stromal cells' by others. (Pap HP ThinPrep®)

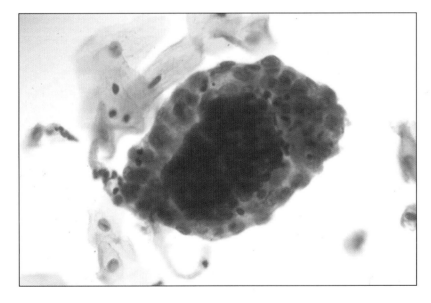

Figure 2.23

Exodus

A cluster of endometrial cells with tightly packed hyperchromatic stromal cells in the center, surrounded by glandular cells with more cytoplasm. Note that the glandular cell nuclei lie parallel to the edge of the cluster, unlike those of endocervical cell nuclei, which are always perpendicular to the edge. (Pap HP ThinPrep®)

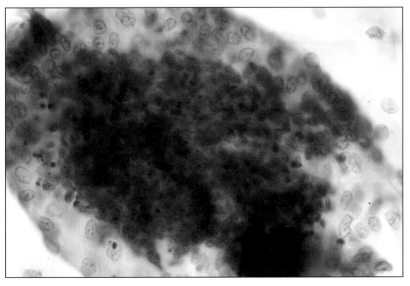

Figure 2.24

Exodus

In the SurePath® preparation the exodus shows similar features, with crowded dark central stromal cells and peripheral glandular cells. Note the copious cytoplasm, variable nuclear size, and irregular nuclei of the glandular cells. (Pap HP SurePath®)

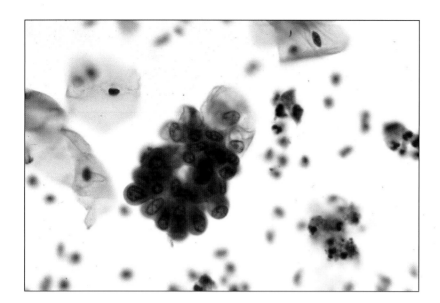

Figure 2.25

Endometrial cells (IUD changes)

A cluster of hyperchromatic endometrial cells, some with enlarged nuclei and abundant cytoplasm. (Pap HP SurePath®)

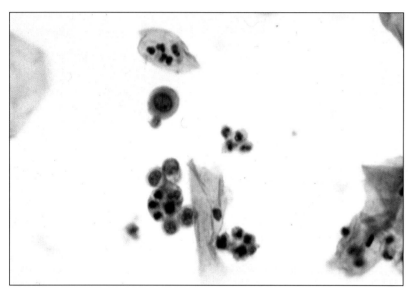

Figure 2.26

Endometrial cells (IUD changes)

The cluster of vacuolated endometrial cells has some nuclei larger than the surrounding neutrophils, and prominent nucleoli. There is a single very large endometrial cell at 12 o'clock. (Pap HP ThinPrep®)

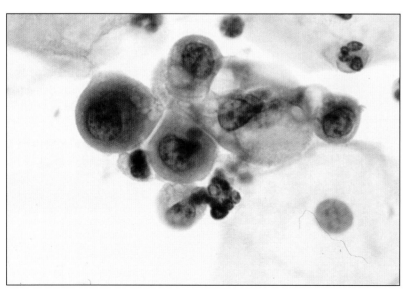

Figure 2.27

Endometrial cells (IUD changes)

These atypical vacuolated endometrial cells display hyperchromatic nuclei, one much larger than the adjacent neutrophils and intermediate cell nucleus. (Pap OI Conventional smear)

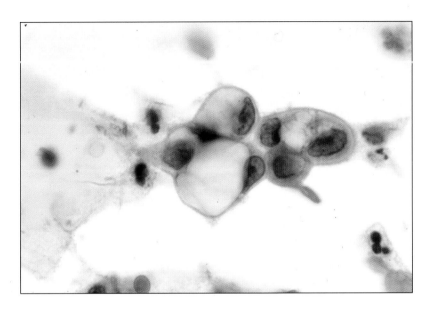

Figure 2.28

Endometrial cells (IUD changes)

A cluster of endometrial cells with nucleoli and large cytoplasmic vacuoles. These features may even suggest a neoplastic process in an older woman if clinical details are not available. (Pap HP Conventional smear)

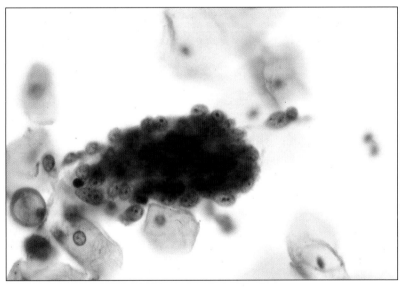

Figure 2.29

Endometriosis

This cluster of small glandular cells displays prominent nucleoli and looks atypical. It can be misdiagnosed as glandular neoplasia. (Pap HP SurePath®)

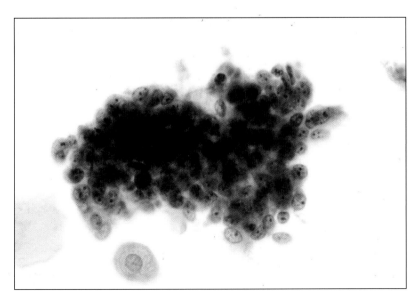

Figure 2.30

Endometriosis

This image is from the same smear as Figure 2.29. In this cluster of cells with prominent nucleoli there is a suggestion of smaller, darker cells in the center, resembling the pattern of exodus. (Pap HP SurePath®)

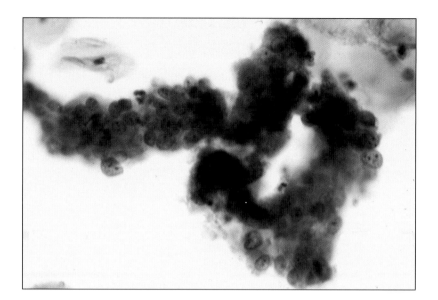

Figure 2.31

Endometriosis

Elongated crowded clusters of atypical glandular cells with small nucleoli are seen here. These can appear suspicious for endocervical adenocarcinoma *in situ*. (Pap HP SurePath®)

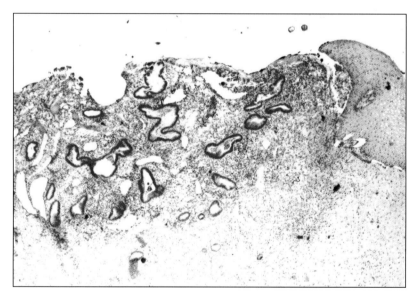

Figure 2.32

Endometriosis

This is the cervical biopsy of the case displaying the abnormal cells above, showing endometriosis. (H&E HP)

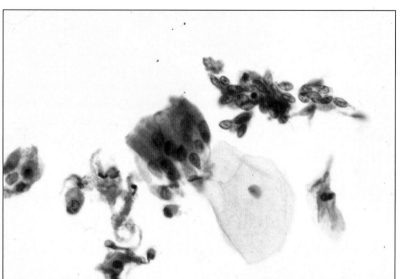

Figure 2.33

Reserve cells

A cluster of reserve cells with spindled nuclei and no visible cytoplasm is seen adjacent to the endocervical cells in the center of the field. These two types of cells are often seen together as reserve cells in a Pap smear are indicative of endocervical reserve cell hyperplasia. (Pap HP ThinPrep®)

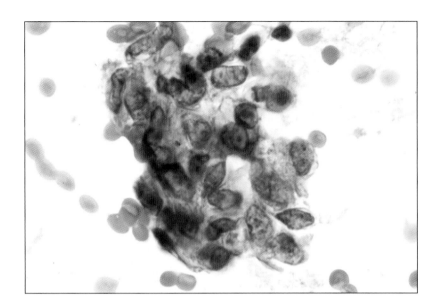

Figure 2.34

Reserve cells

This is a loose cluster of cells with elongated nuclei, vesicular chromatin, and incomplete cytoplasm. (Pap HP Comventional smear)

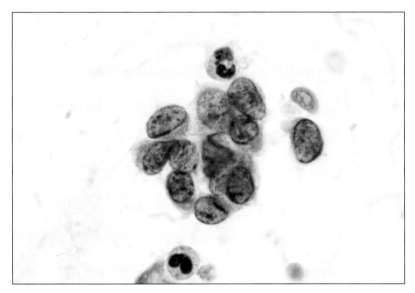

Figure 2.35

Reserve cells

Groups of small cells (nuclei the size of polymorphs), with smooth ovoid nuclei, slightly granular chromatin, and a tiny amount of cytoplasm are seen in this field. (Pap OI Conventional smear)

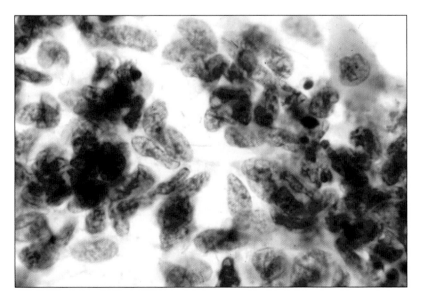

Figure 2.36

Reserve cells

This is a collection of cells with spindle-shaped to ovoid nuclei and vesicular chromatin. The cytoplasm is not clearly visualized. Reserve cells are usually accompanied by endocervical cells (see Figure 2.33). These are not endometrial cells, although some have referred to them as 'endometrial stromal cells'. Note the immature squamous metaplastic cell in the top right corner. (Pap OI Conventional smear)

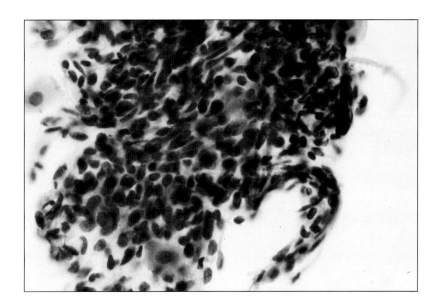

Figure 2.37

Lower uterine segment

A tight cluster of small glandular cells from the lower uterine segment admixed with elongated stromal cell nuclei. The cells that originate in the lower uterine segment resemble endocervical cells in tight sheets, but also resemble endometrial cells, as they are cuboidal and often are admixed with spindle-shaped stromal cells. (Pap HP SurePath®)

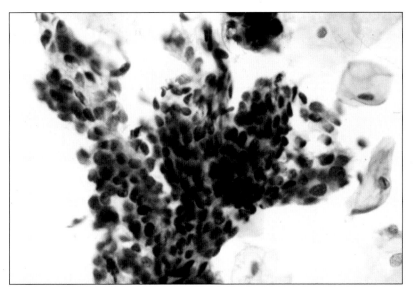

Figure 2.38

Lower uterine segment

This ThinPrep® shows similar features to Figure 2.37. The glandular cells are crowded and some elongated stromal cells are seen at 12 o'clock and 6 o'clock. (Pap HP ThinPrep®)

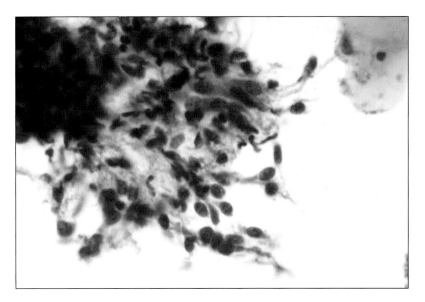

Figure 2.39

Lower uterine segment

As noted in Figures 2.37 and 2.38, this is represented by overlapping groups of small glandular cells accompanied by spindle-shaped stromal cells as seen here. (Pap LP ThinPrep®)

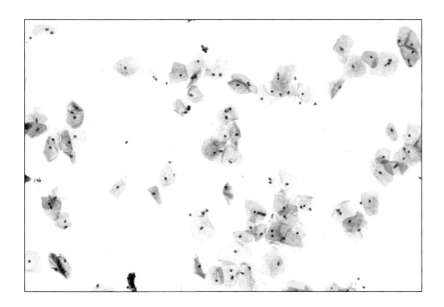

Figure 3.4

Early luteal phase

Intermediate cells predominate in this smear, taken in the early luteal phase. Note the clean background seen in the ThinPrep® smear. (Pap LP ThinPrep®)

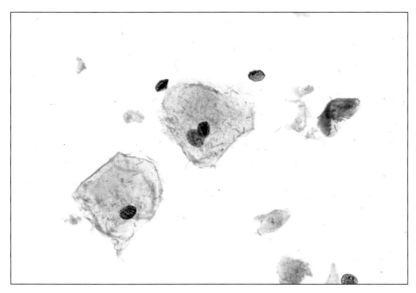

Figure 3.5

Cytolysis

Two intermediate cells are seen here with small cytoplasmic remnants and bare intermediate cell nuclei in the background. Cytolysis occurs during the luteal phase of the cycle when, under the influence of progesterone, intermediate cells containing glycogen abound, providing nourishment for lactobacilli (Doderlein bacilli). Cytolysis is also noted during the later part of pregnancy and in early menopause, again associated with lack of estrogen and prevalence of progesterone. (Pap HP ThinPrep®)

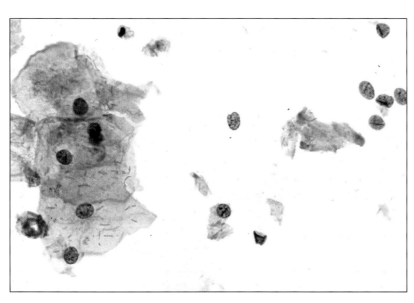

Figure 3.6

Cytolysis

Note the rod-shaped Doderlein bacilli overlying the intermediate cells on the left. Cytoplasmic remnants and bare intermediate cell nuclei are also seen. These small bare nuclei should not be confused with the large abnormal bare nuclei associated with severe dysplasia (see Figures 6.27 and 6.28). (Pap OI ThinPrep®)

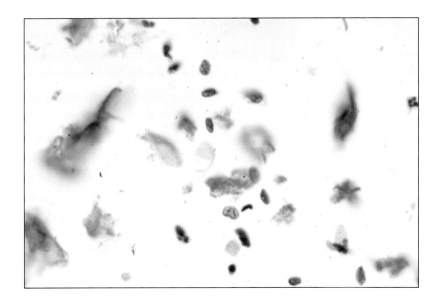

Figure 3.7

Cytolysis

Bare intermediate cell nuclei and cytoplasmic remnants are seen on different planes due to the nature of this preparation. Note the variability in size of the bare intermediate cell nuclei. This precludes the use of large bare nuclei as clues to severe dysplasia in SurePath® smears. (Pap HP SurePath®)

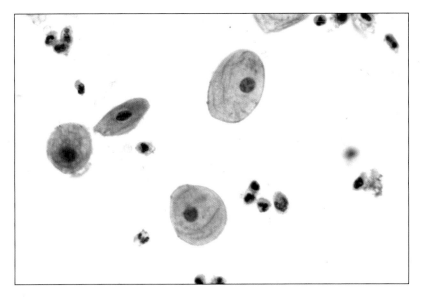

Figure 3.8

Postpartum smear pattern

In this field, there are only parabasal cells and a few neutrophil polymorphs. (Pap LP ThinPrep®)

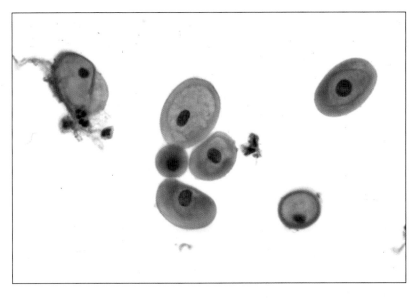

Figure 3.9

Postpartum smear pattern

Postpartum smears show an atrophic pattern due to lack of circulating estrogen. Note the parabasal cells in this field. (Pap HP SurePath®)

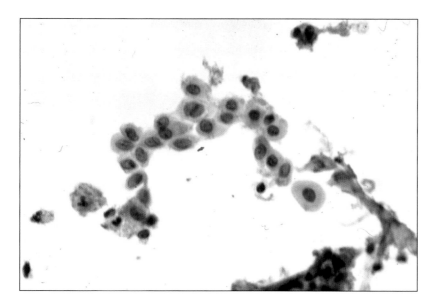

Figure 3.10

Postmenopausal smear pattern

This illustrates small immature parabasal cells with a high nuclear : cytoplasmic ratio. These parabasal cells are much smaller than those usually seen in postpartum smears. (Pap HP ThinPrep®)

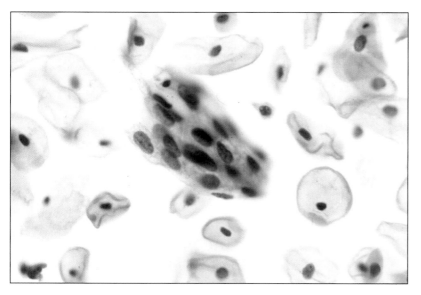

Figure 3.11

Postmenopausal smear pattern

In the center of the field is a cluster of parabasal cells with a high nuclear : cytoplasmic ratio. The single parabasal cells in the background are slightly more mature, with more cytoplasm and smaller nuclei. (Pap HP SurePath®)

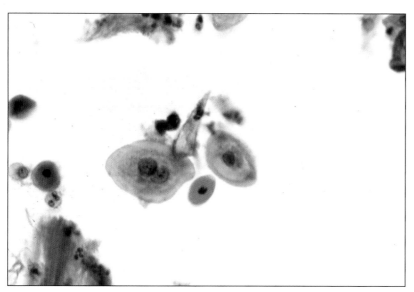

Figure 3.12

Postmenopausal smear pattern

In this field, there is a small keratinized cell below the larger parabasal cells. Small keratinized cells are not uncommonly seen in postmenopausal Pap smears. (Pap HP ThinPrep®)

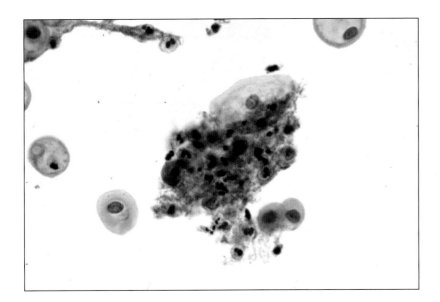

Figure 3.13

Atrophic vaginitis

Note that polymorphs clump in this preparation, and therefore the parabasal cells are still clearly visualized. (Pap HP ThinPrep®)

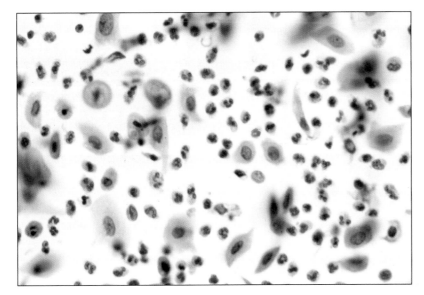

Figure 3.14

Atrophic vaginitis

Single parabasal cells are seen here scattered among the polymorphs. (Pap HP SurePath®)

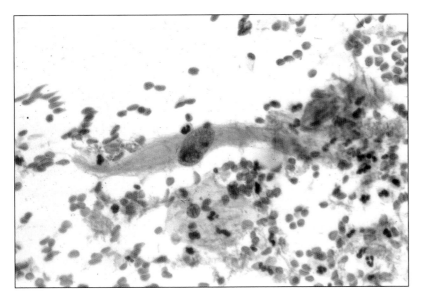

Figure 3.15

Decidual change

Conventional smear showing a large cell with abundant cytoplasm and an enlarged nucleus with a nucleolus. There is evidence of cytolysis and there are red blood cells in the background. (Pap HP Conventional smear)

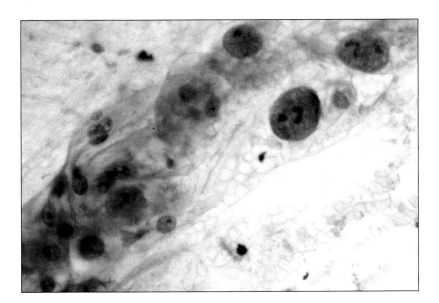

Figure 3.16

Decidual change

This is a field from a conventional smear showing cells with enlarged, hyperchromatic but smooth-bordered nuclei with nucleoli. Decidual change can mimic dysplasia but dysplastic cells do not exhibit nucleoli. (Pap HP Conventional smear)

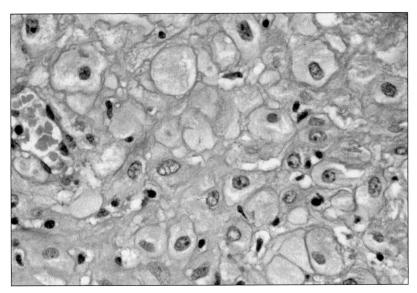

Figure 3.17

Decidualized polyp

This biopsy is from the same patient as in Figure 3.16, showing a decidualized polyp with cells similar to those seen in the Pap smear. (H&E HP)

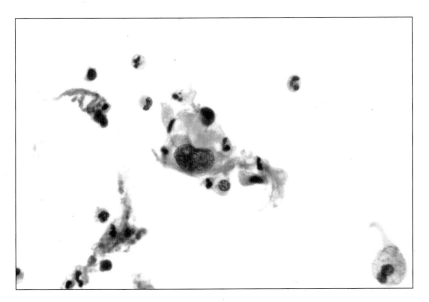

Figure 3.18

Decidual change

Note the cell with an enlarged hyperchromatic nucleus. This would be suggestive of dysplasia if there was further evidence in the rest of the smear but the history of pregnancy and the absence of further abnormality is indicative of decidual change. However, if doubt persists, the smear should be reported as atypical squamous cells of undetermined significance (ASC-US). (Pap HP ThinPrep®)

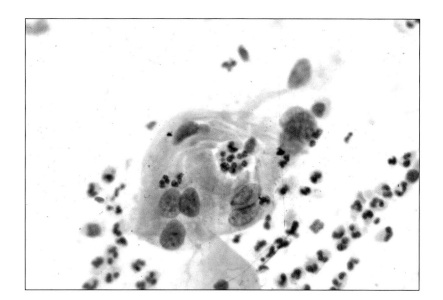

Figure 3.19

Decidual change

Cells with abundant cytoplasm and enlarged but bland nuclei are seen in this conventional smear from a pregnant woman. (Pap HP Conventional smear)

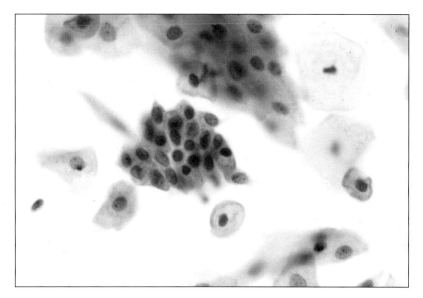

Figure 3.20

Endocervical-like cells

In this SurePath® vaginal smear from a post-hysterectomy patient, there is a sheet of endocervical-like cells with somewhat delicate cytoplasm in the center of the field. Similarly, metaplastic-like cells may be noted in such smears. (Pap HP SurePath®)

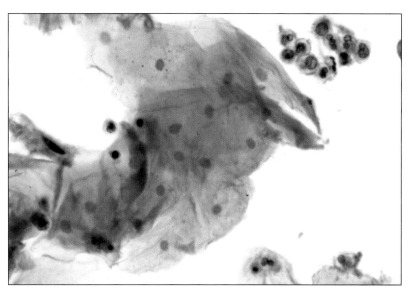

Figure 3.21

Karyolysis

The nuclei in these intermediate cells are undergoing degenerative changes and appear to be dissolving out of the cells. This pattern is often seen in vaginal smears. Anucleate squames (see Figure 1.21) are also common in vaginal smears. (Pap HP ThinPrep®)

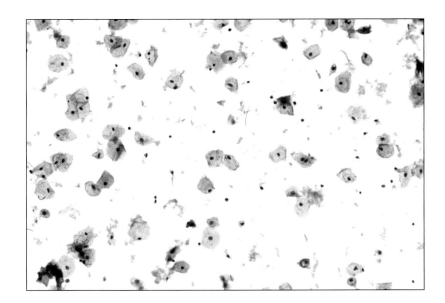

Figure 3.22

Red blood cells

The ThinPrep® process lyses red blood cells. In this field lysed erythrocytes form small clumps that do not obscure the epithelial cells. Any material other than epithelial cells tends to form clumps with this preparation (e.g. polymorphs, debris, and tumor diathesis). (Pap LP ThinPrep®)

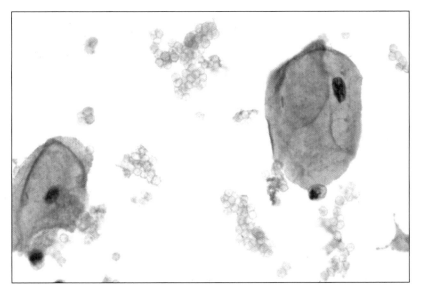

Figure 3.23

Red blood cells

When abundant blood is present in the specimen, red blood cells are seen as clumps of ghost or empty cells in ThinPrep® smears. (Pap HP ThinPrep®)

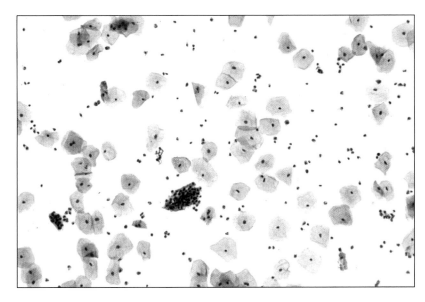

Figure 3.24

Neutrophil polymorphs

In ThinPrep® smears, polymorphs do not obscure the epithelial cell population as they lie in the background singly or form small clumps. (Pap LP ThinPrep®)

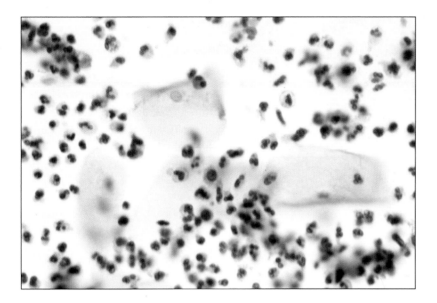

Figure 3.25

Neutrophil polymorphs

Polymorphs are not normally present in SurePath® smears. However, when they are present in abundance, they are distributed throughout the smear and may also overlie the squamous cells as seen here. (Pap HP SurePath®)

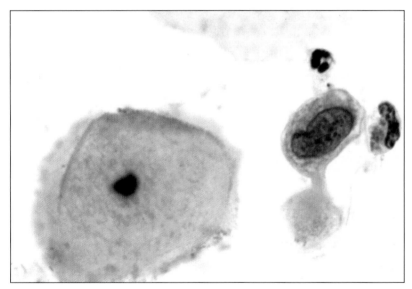

Figure 3.26

Histiocyte

Note the histiocyte with its bean-shaped nucleus and delicate cytoplasm adjacent to the superficial cell. Single histiocytes can sometimes mimic high grade squamous intraepithelial lesion (HSIL) cells. (Pap OI ThinPrep®)

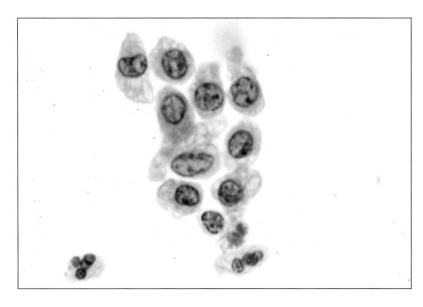

Figure 3.27

Histiocyte

Histiocytes in Pap smears are variable in size. Here, they are small, the size of neutrophils. (Pap HP ThinPrep®)

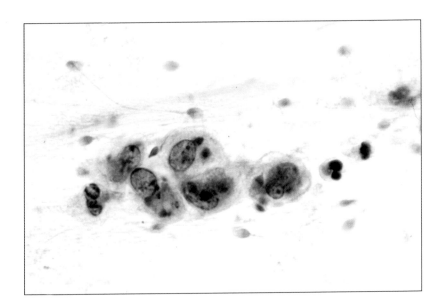

Figure 3.28

Histiocytes

Histiocytes act as scavengers. Here, the histiocytes show phagocytosed spermatozoa. (Pap HP Conventional smear)

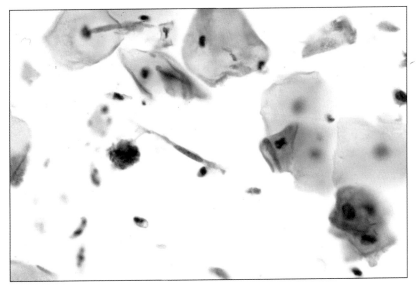

Figure 3.29

Fibroblast

The thin spindle-shaped cell in the center of the field is a fibroblast (distinguished from fiber cells of invasive carcinoma by the fact that the nucleus does not cause the cytoplasm to bulge). These may be seen in varying numbers following a variety of procedures, including biopsy. (Pap HP SurePath®)

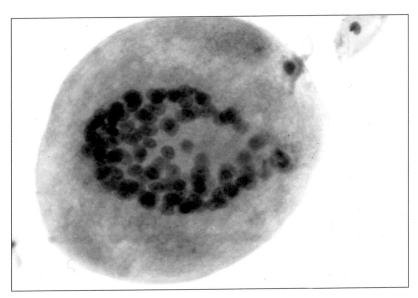

Figure 3.30

Multinucleated giant histiocyte

This is a multinucleated histiocyte in a ThinPrep® smear. These giant cells are most commonly seen in postmenopausal smears but may also be noted in postpartum Pap smears. (Pap HP ThinPrep®)

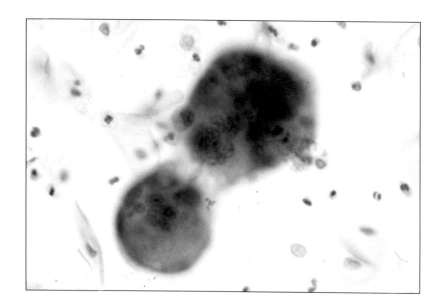

Figure 3.31

Multinucleated giant histiocyte

This is a large dumb-bell-shaped multinucleated histiocyte in a SurePath® smear, a cell that is usually seen in atrophic smears. (Pap HP SurePath®)

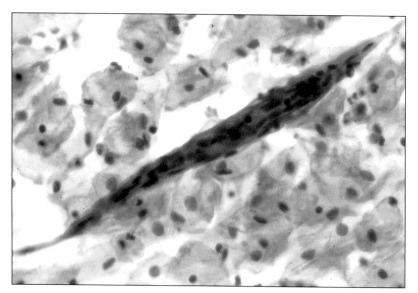

Figure 3.32

Parakeratosis

This is a conventional smear showing a sharp spike, composed of keratinized squamous cells with degenerating nuclei. (Pap HP Conventional smear)

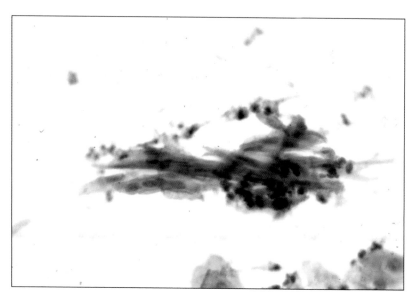

Figure 3.33

Parakeratosis

A clump of parakeratotic cells with degenerative nuclear changes is seen in this field. (Pap HP ThinPrep®)

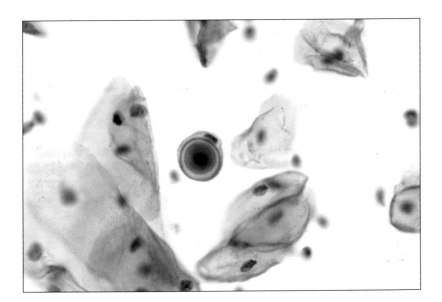

Figure 3.34

Squamous pearl

This is a benign squamous pearl consisting of a tight whorl of squamous cells. (Pap HP SurePath®)

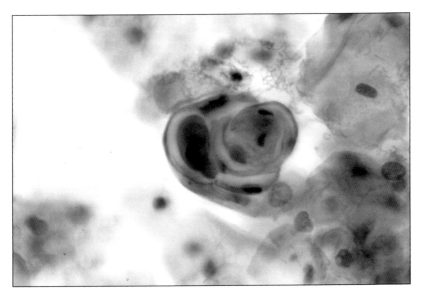

Figure 3.35

Squamous pearl

A tight cluster of squamous cells forming a pearl is seen in this conventional smear. (Pap HP Conventional smear)

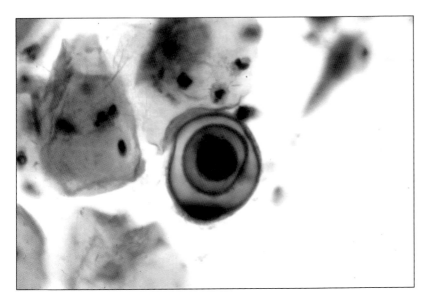

Figure 3.36

Squamous pearl

Another squamous pearl. (Pap HP Conventional smear)

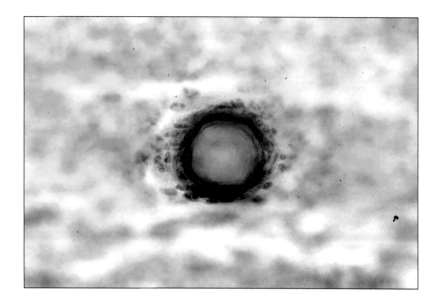

Figure 3.37

Psammoma body

This is a conventional smear showing a laminated psammoma body. A careful search should be made for the presence of abnormal glandular cells when a psammoma body is noted in the smear, although they are not always a sinister finding. No abnormal cells were present in this smear. (Pap HP Conventional smear)

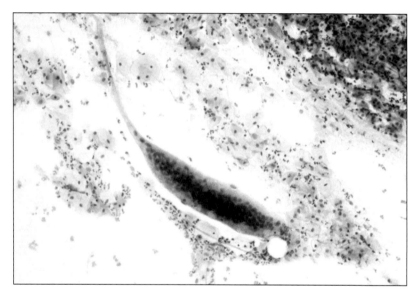

Figure 3.38

Syncytiotrophoblast

This field from a conventional smear shows an enormous elongated cell with multiple nuclei, representing a synctiotrophoblast. These are seen in postpartum smears. (Pap LP Conventional smear)

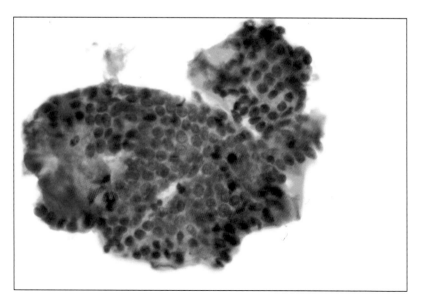

Figure 3.39

Neovagina colonic epithelium

This sheet of uniform glandular cells is derived from the colonic epithelium obtained from a neovagina constructed from colon. (Pap HP ThinPrep®)

Recommended reading

1. Chhieng DC, Elgert P, Cangiarella JF, Cohen JM. Significance of AGUS Pap smears in pregnant and postpartum women. *Acta Cytol* 2001;**45**:294–9.
2. Rhatigan RM. Endocervical gland atypia secondary to Arias-Stella change. *Arch Pathol Lab Med* 1992;**116**:943–6.
3. Kobayashi TK, Okamoto H. Cytopathology of pregnancy-induced cell patterns in cervicovaginal smears. *Am J Clin Pathol* 2000;**114**:S6–20.
4. Michael CW, Esfahani FM. Pregnancy-related changes: a retrospective review of 278 cervical smears. *Diagn Cytopathol* 1997;**17**:99–107.
5. Schnreider C, Barnes LA. Ectopic decidual reaction of the uterine cervix: frequency and cytologic presentation. *Acta Cytol* 1981;**25**:616–22.
6. Benoit JL, Kini SR. "Arias-Stella reaction"-like changes in endocervical glandular epithelium in cervical smears during pregnancy and postpartum states – a potential diagnostic pitfall. *Diagn Cytopathol* 1996;**14**:349–55.
7. Mulvany NJ, Khan A, Ostor A. Arias-Stella reaction associated with cervical pregnancy. Report of a case with a cytologic presentation. *Acta Cytol* 1994;**38**:218–22.
8. Pisharodi LR, Jovanoska S. Spectrum of cytologic changes in pregnancy. A review of 100 abnormal cervicovaginal smears, with emphasis on diagnostic pitfalls. *Acta Cytol* 1995;**39**:905–8.
9. Possover M, Drahonowski J, Plaul K, Schneider A. Laparoscopic-assisted formation of a colon neovagina. *Surg Endosc* 2001;**15**:623.
10. Motoyama S, Laoag-Fernandez JB, Mochizuki S, et al. Vaginoplasty with Interceed absorbable adhesion barrier for complete squamous epithelialization in vaginal agenesis. *Am J Obstet Gynecol* 2003;**185**:1260–4.
11. Steiner E, Woernle F, Kuhn W, et al. Carcinoma of the neovagina: case report and review of the literature. *Gynecol Oncol* 2002;**84**:171–5.
12. Holmquist ND, Bellina JH, Danos ML. Vaginal and cervical cytologic changes following laser treatment. *Acta Cytol* 1976;**20**:290–4.

4 Benign disorders of the cervix

Inflammation, reactive changes and repair

Inflammatory changes in squamous cells include slight nuclear enlargement (up to twice the size of an intermediate cell nucleus), bi- or multinucleation, a small perinuclear halo, and abundant neutrophil polymorphs in the background. Reactive changes comprise slight nuclear enlargement as with inflammation in squamous cells, and multinucleation with prominent nucleoli in endocervical and metaplastic cells. The chromatin may appear granular or evenly coarse. The changes of repair are an exaggeration of reactive changes in endocervical or squamous metaplastic cells, with variably sized nuclei, bi- or multinucleation, prominent nucleoli, and ingestion of neutrophil polymorphs. The clusters of cells appear 'pulled-out' in conventional smears, but are more rounded in liquid-based smears.

Infections and organisms

Infections are usually accompanied by acute inflammatory cells and histiocytes, with proteinaceous material in the background. Certain infections display clues, such as pink staining of most of the squamous cells and perinuclear haloes with Trichomonas infection. With Candida, too, there is often marked inflammation in the background with reactive cellular changes including nuclear enlargement and phagocytosed neutrophils. Leptothrix is a commensal, which usually accompanies *Trichomonas vaginilis*. Clue cells are evidence of Gardnerella infection and are reported as showing a shift in vaginal flora consistent with bacterial vaginosis. Herpes simplex virus infection shows typical cellular changes including giant cells with multinucleation, nuclear molding, and 'ground-glass' chromatin. It is also accompanied by inflamed and reactive endocervical cells, often with abundant polymorphs. Acintomyces-like organisms do not always induce inflammatory changes in cells.

Other cellular changes

Radiation to the pelvic area shows long-term effects lasting for decades. The squamous cells have bizarre shapes, with enlargement of both the cell and the nucleus; therefore the nuclear:cytoplasmic ratio is normal. Amphophilia is common. Radiation changes include numerous neutrophil polymorphs and multinucleated giant histiocytes, especially soon after treatment. Nucleoli are commonly seen, as well as degenerative changes. Chemotherapy also causes cellular changes, usually in the form of nuclear enlargement with smudged chromatin.

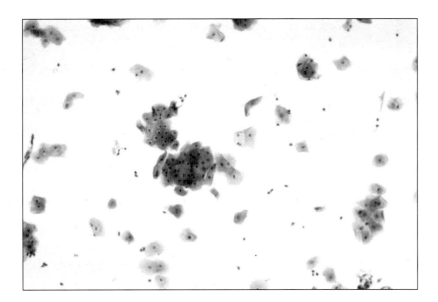

Figure 4.1

Inflammatory changes

This view shows inflammatory perinuclear haloes, visible even on low power. A few polymorphs are seen in the background. The pink appearance of the cells should prompt a careful search for *Trichomonas vaginalis*. (Pap LP ThinPrep®)

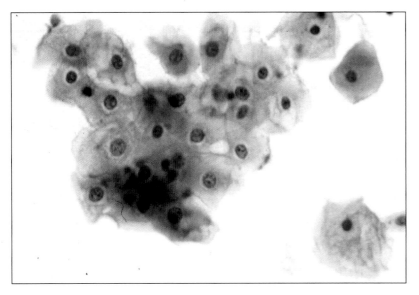

Figure 4.2

Inflammatory changes

This high power view shows a sheet of squamous cells with slightly enlarged nuclei, perinuclear haloes, and reactive nuclei. The perinuclear haloes of inflammation are much smaller than those of human papillomavirus (HPV) change and are not accompanied by abnormal nuclei or a thickened rim of cytoplasm. Margination of the chromatin (i.e. a thick rim of heterochromatin around the nuclear margin), is a common feature of inflammation. (Pap HP ThinPrep®)

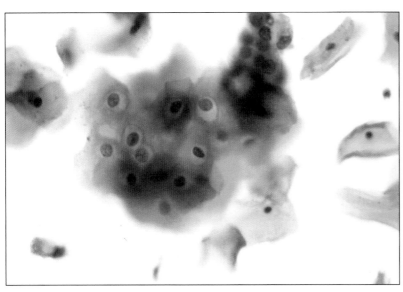

Figure 4.3

Inflammatory changes

Note the small perinuclear haloes in the cluster of squamous cells, indicative of inflammation. (Pap HP SurePath®)

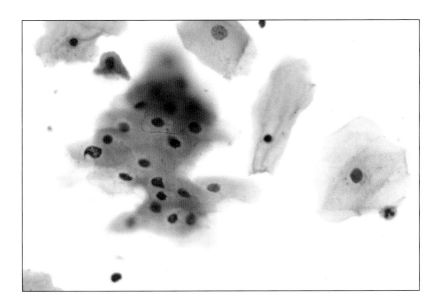

Figure 4.4

Inflammatory changes

The cluster shows indistinct perinuclear haloes as well as degenerative nuclear changes in the form of spiky irregularities and smudged chromatin. Nuclear margin irregularities are seen in degeneration, accompanying other features, such as pyknosis and indistinct chromatin. (Pap HP SurePath®)

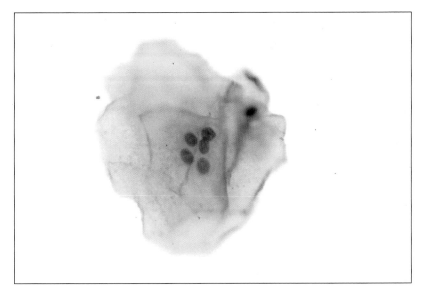

Figure 4.5

Reactive changes

This somewhat folded superficial cell has five small nuclei and no perinuclear halo, suggesting reactive rather than inflammatory changes. (Pap HP ThinPrep®)

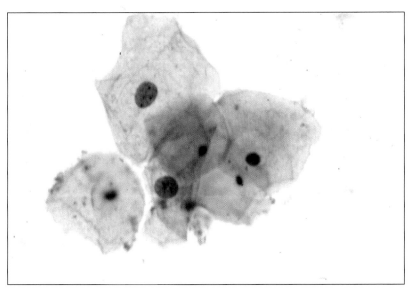

Figure 4.6

Reactive changes

Two of these cells show nuclear enlargement about twice the size of the intermediate cell nucleus at 3 o'clock. The nuclear margins are smooth and their chromatin is bland. This nuclear enlargement can be interpreted as due to reactive changes. There are no perinuclear haloes. (Pap HP ThinPrep®)

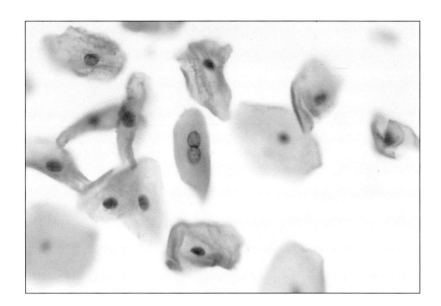

Figure 4.7

Reactive changes

Note the binucleated squamous cell in the center of the field. Binucleation often accompanies inflammatory changes but in this case there are no perinuclear haloes or accompanying polymorphs to suggest inflammation. (Pap LP SurePath®)

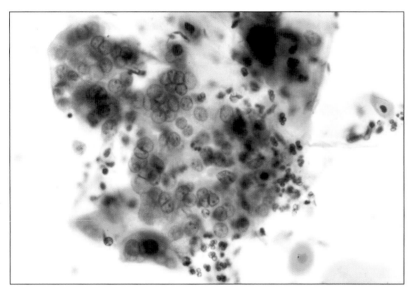

Figure 4.8

Reactive endocervical cells

The endocervical cells seen here are multinucleated and contain small nucleoli. Note the neutrophil polymorphs in the background. (Pap HP SurePath®)

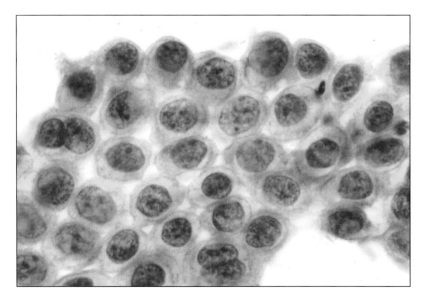

Figure 4.9

Reactive endocervical cells

This high power view is of endocervical cells showing reactive changes in the form of granular chromatin visible nucleoli and occasional binucleation. More chromatin detail than usual is seen under oil immersion. (Pap OI ThinPrep®)

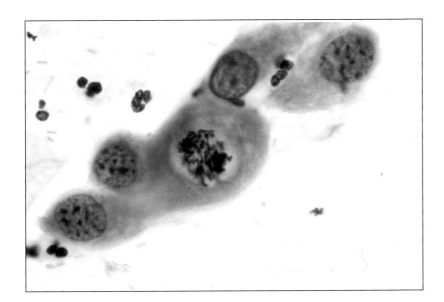

Figure 4.10

Reactive endocervical cells

This is a group of endocervical cells showing marked nuclear enlargement (4–5 times the size of the polymorphs in the field), hyperchromasia, and a mitotic figure. Reactive changes often appear worse than glandular neoplasia. (Pap OI ThinPrep®)

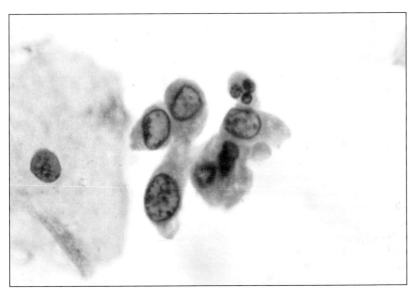

Figure 4.11

Reactive endocervical cells

These endocervical cells show nuclear enlargement and coarser chromatin than usual. Note the polymorph for nuclear size comparison. This appearance can be mistaken for high grade squamous intraepithelial lesion (HSIL), though in this case the patient had an endocervical polyp. (Pap HP ThinPrep®)

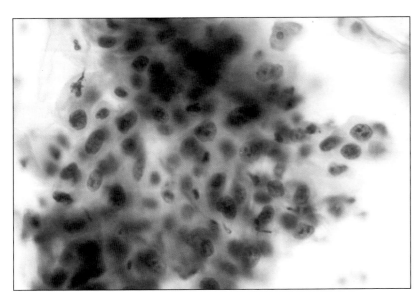

Figure 4.12

Reactive endocervical cells

This sheet of endocervical cells shows prominent nucleoli and nuclei of varying sizes. Note also the abundant cytoplasm which is quite frequently seen in endocervical cells in SurePath® smears. This may lead to difficulty distinguishing endocervical from metaplastic cells in these preparations. (Pap HP SurePath®)

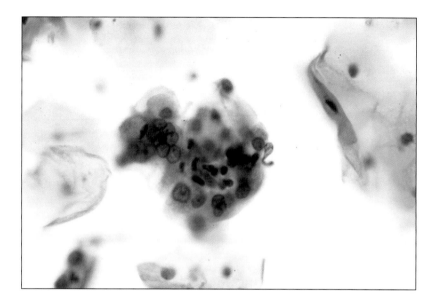

Figure 4.13

Reactive endocervical cells

Multinucleated reactive endocervical cells are seen here. Some of the cells show enlarged nuclei and nucleoli. (Pap HP SurePath®)

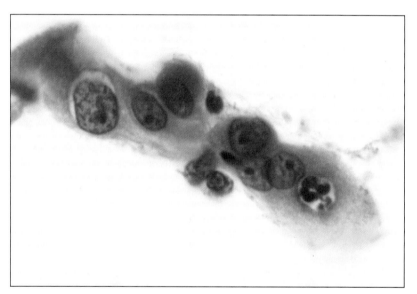

Figure 4.14

Reactive squamous metaplastic cells

Metaplastic cells showing multinucleation and prominent nucleoli. Note the engulfed polymorph. These changes are bordering on repair. (Pap HP ThinPrep®)

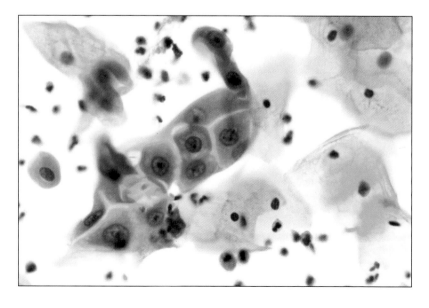

Figure 4.15

Reactive/reparative change in metaplastic cells

This is a sheet of squamous metaplastic cells showing prominent nucleoli. (Pap HP SurePath®)

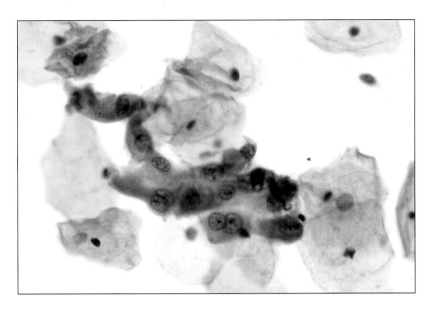

Figure 4.16

Repair

Note the sheet of endocervical/ metaplastic cells showing nuclear enlargement, prominent nucleoli, and phagocytosis of polymorphs. These groups are often rounded in liquid-based preparations, unlike the typical 'pulled-out' appearance in conventional smears. (Pap HP ThinPrep®)

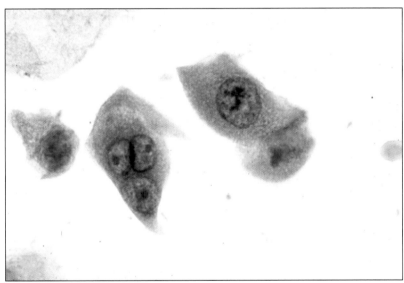

Figure 4.17

Repair

Squamous metaplastic cells showing reactive/reparative changes with multinucleation and prominent nucleoli. Note that the nuclear margin remains round and smooth. (Pap OI ThinPrep®)

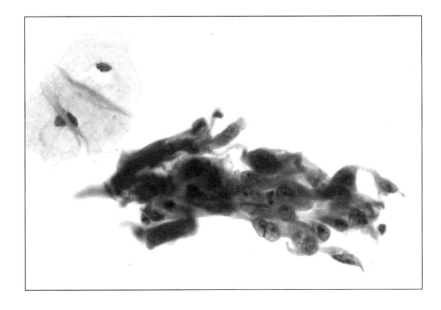

Figure 4.18

Repair

Occasionally in ThinPrep® smears, repair is represented by 'pulled-out' sheets of squamous metaplastic/endocervical cells with binucleation, nuclear enlargement, and prominent nuclei as seen in this figure. (Pap HP ThinPrep®)

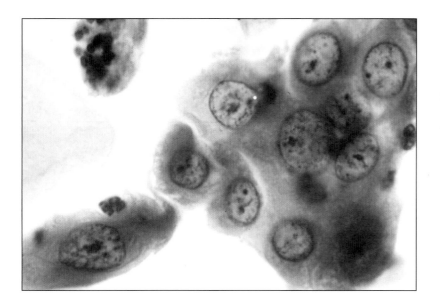

Figure 4.19

Repair

Here, the sheet of endocervical cells shows round, enlarged, variably sized nuclei, and prominent nucleoli. (Pap OI ThinPrep®)

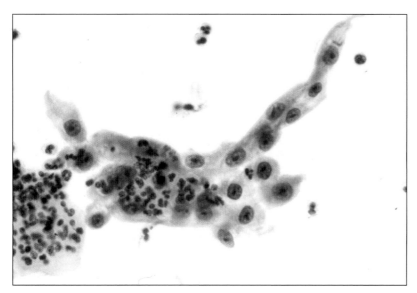

Figure 4.20

Repair

A 'pulled-out' sheet of metaplastic cells with prominent nucleoli and phagocytosed neutrophil polymorphs. This is the pattern seen in conventional smears. (Pap HP ThinPrep®)

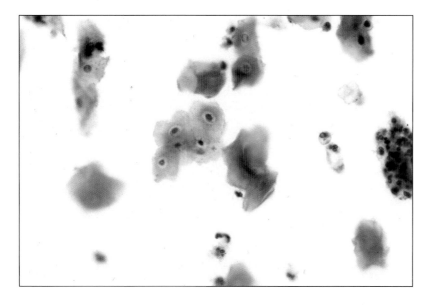

Figure 4.21

Trichomomas vaginalis

This appearance with predominantly pink-staining cells and perinuclear inflammatory haloes should alert one to the possibility of Trichomomas, although the organisms are not clearly visualized in this field. (Pap LP ThinPrep®)

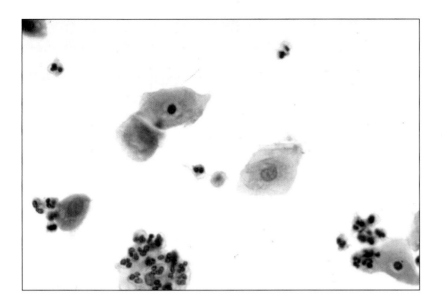

Figure 4.22

Trichomomas vaginalis

Note the organism in the center of the field, about the size of a polymorph but clearly distinguishable from the polymorphs in the background. The extent of the inflammatory changes varies with the size of the organism, from severe inflammation with small trichomonads to no inflammation whatsoever in the presence of larger organisms. (Professor E. Wachtel, personal communication) (Pap HP ThinPrep®)

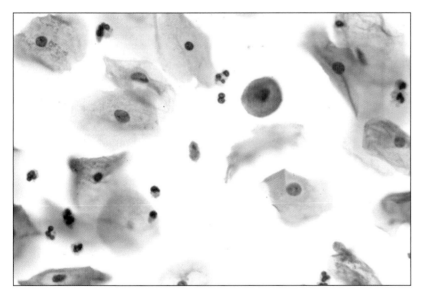

Figure 4.23

Trichomonas vaginalis

The squamous cells are pink-staining. Note the trichomonad in the center of the field. The pink intermediate cell to the right of the trichomonad shows a faint perinuclear halo. (Pap HP SurePath®)

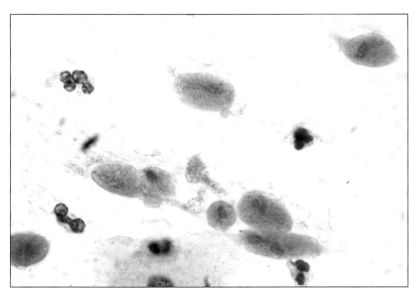

Figure 4.24

Trichomonas vaginalis

The organisms vary in size, are usually pear-shaped with an elongated nucleus, and often show pink-staining granules. (Pap OI Conventional smear)

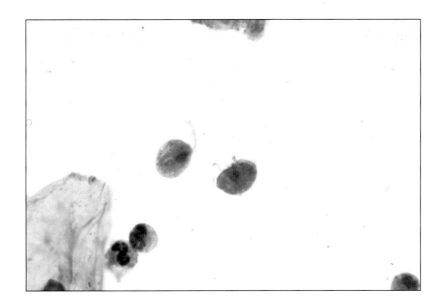

Figure 4.25

Trichomonas vaginalis

Two trichomonads, one of which has a flagellum, are seen in this field. (Pap OI ThinPrep®)

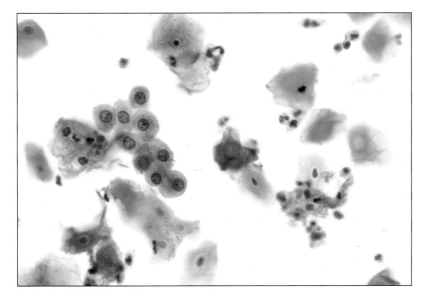

Figure 4.26

Trichomonas vaginalis

This field shows a group of squamous metaplastic cells, some cells showing inflammatory haloes, and a few organisms in the clump of debris at 4 o'clock. (Pap LP ThinPrep®)

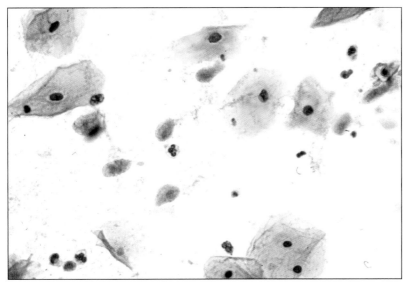

Figure 4.27

Trichomonas vaginalis

This image shows organisms that are 2–3 times the size of polymorphs. (Pap OI Conventional smear)

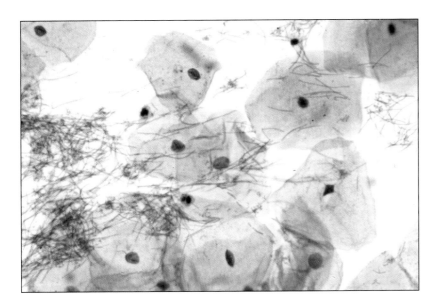

Figure 4.28

Leptothrix

These long filamentous organisms are seen overlying squamous cells in this field. They are commensals and often accompany *Trichomonas vaginalis*. (Pap HP ThinPrep®)

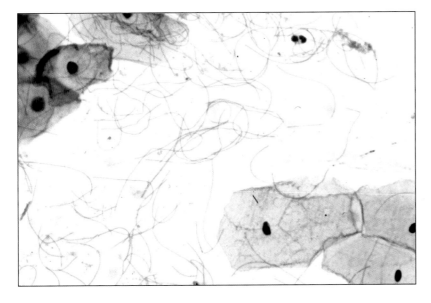

Figure 4.29

Leptothrix

These organisms can be extremely long and on conventional smears look like a child's scribbles. (Pap HP Conventional smear)

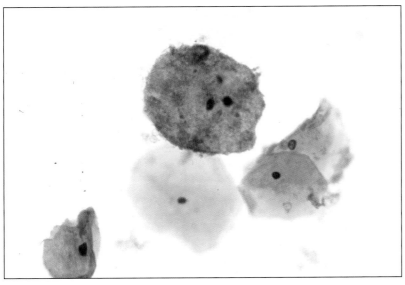

Figure 4.30

Clue cells

The epithelial cell in the center is covered by coccobacilli while the background is clear. Formerly referred to as *Hemophilus vaginalis,* then as *Gardnerella*, this appearance is now reported as coccobacilli consistent with a shift in vaginal flora suggesting bacterial vaginosis. (Pap OI ThinPrep®)

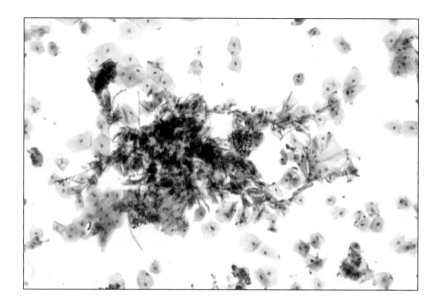

Figure 4.31

Candida

The central cluster of cells appears to be skewered by Candida hyphae. This 'kebab'-like appearance is typical of this organism. The pseudohyphae stain pink in conventional smears but often stain blue in liquid-based Pap smears. (Pap LP ThinPrep®)

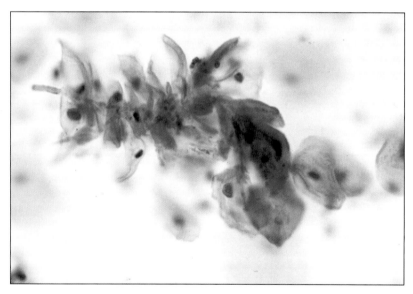

Figure 4.32

Candida

The 'skewered' appearance is also noted in SurePath® smears. Here, too, the hyphae are blue rather than pink. (Pap HP SurePath®)

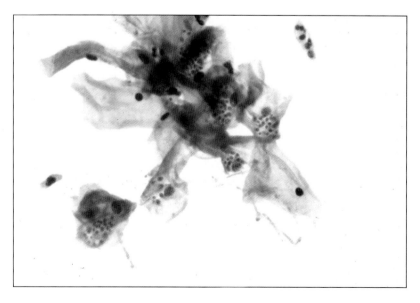

Figure 4.33

Candida

This field shows clumps of Candida spores overlying mature squamous cells. (Pap HP ThinPrep®)

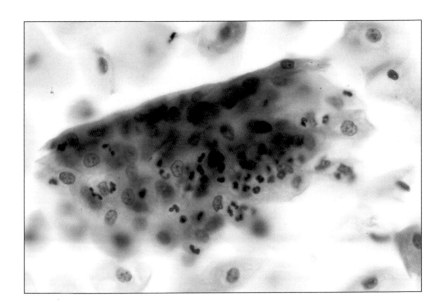

Figure 4.34

Candida

This SurePath® preparation shows a cluster of cells with reactive nuclear changes, infiltrated by polymorphs. Candida was present elsewhere in the smear. (Pap HP SurePath®)

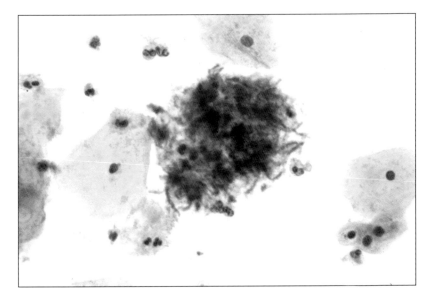

Figure 4.35

Actinomyces-like organisms

These organisms are seen in clumps with central bacillary forms and surrounding filaments. They are associated with intrauterine contraceptive device (IUD) use. In conventional smears, the organisms are sometimes grouped together in a form resembling a brush. (Pap HP ThinPrep®)

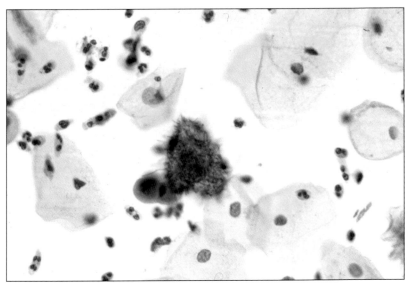

Figure 4.36

Actinomyces-like organisms

The appearance is similar in SurePath® smears, with the bacilli in the center and the filamentous forms at the periphery. (Pap HP SurePath®)

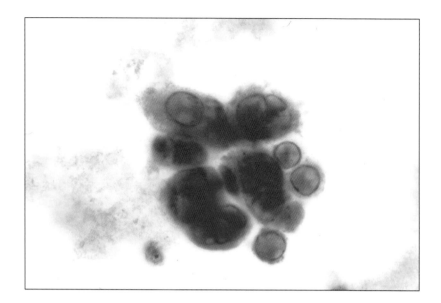

Figure 4.37

Herpes simplex virus

Typically, this infection manifests as multinucleated cells with 'ground-glass' nuclei. (Pap LP ThinPrep®)

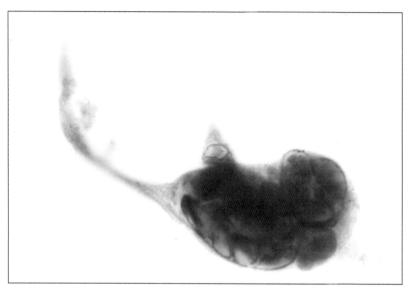

Figure 4.38

Herpes simplex virus

This multinucleated cell shows molded nuclei and 'ground-glass' chromatin, best visualized in the nuclei at the periphery. (Pap OI ThinPrep®)

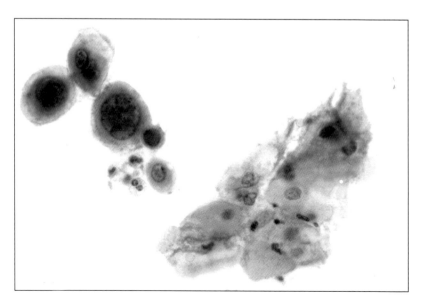

Figure 4.39

Herpes simplex virus

The large abnormal cells on the left show indistinct nuclei with molding and chromatin that has not reached the 'ground-glass' stage. (Pap HP ThinPrep®)

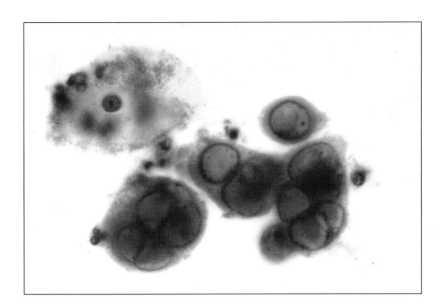

Figure 4.40

Herpes simplex virus

Multinucleation, nuclear molding and 'ground-glass' chromatin are clearly displayed in this ThinPrep® slide. The lack of chromatin detail distinguishes these infected cells from reactive multinucleated endocervical cells. (Pap OI ThinPrep®)

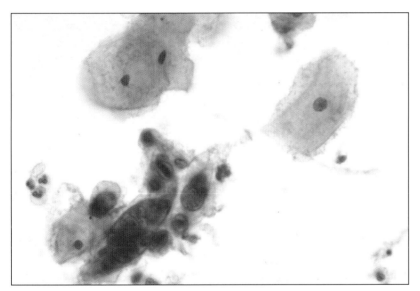

Figure 4.41

Herpes simplex virus

In addition to multinucleation and molding, some intranuclear inclusions are present. (Pap HP ThinPrep®)

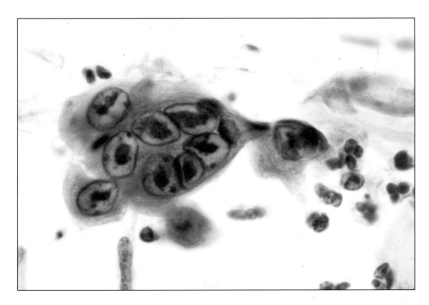

Figure 4.42

Herpes simplex virus

This multinucleated giant cell has enormous intranuclear inclusions. (Pap OI Conventional smear)

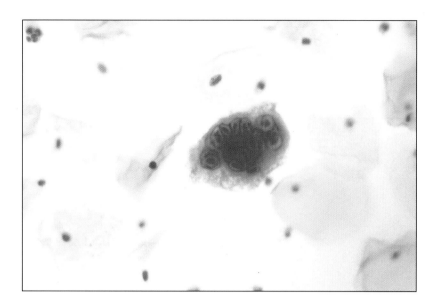

Figure 4.43

Herpes simplex virus

Intranuclear inclusions are clearly visualized in this SurePath® preparation. (Pap OI SurePath®)

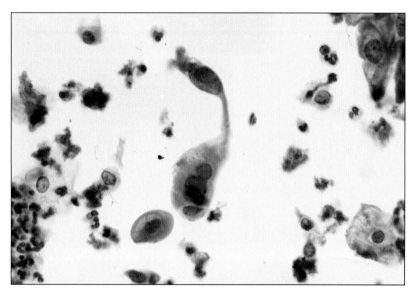

Figure 4.44

Herpes simplex virus

The multinucleated cell in the center of the field has an unusual shape in addition to multinucleation and abnormal chromatin. (Pap HP SurePath®)

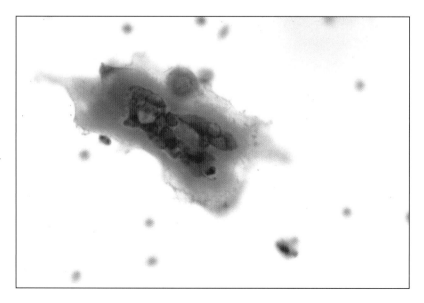

Figure 4.45

Herpes simplex virus

This giant cell displays multinucleation and but may not be recognized as herpes infection because of the abundant cytoplasm. (Pap HP SurePath®)

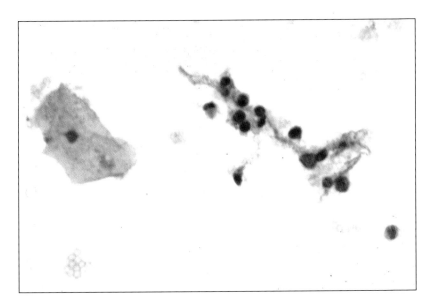

Figure 4.46

Follicular cervicitis

A few lymphoid cells are seen in this field adjacent to an intermediate cell. However, these lymphocytes may be derived from blood as there are clumps of lysed red cells, and ghost red blood cells (lower left corner) in the background. (Pap LP ThinPrep®)

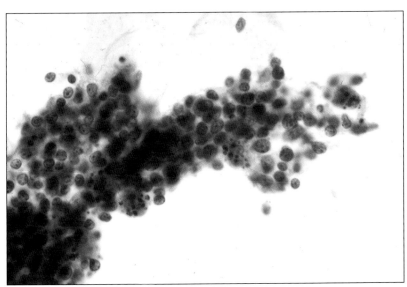

Figure 4.47

Follicular cervicitis

A collection of lymphocytes with admixed histiocytes and several tingible body macrophages, representing a follicle center. (Pap HP ThinPrep®)

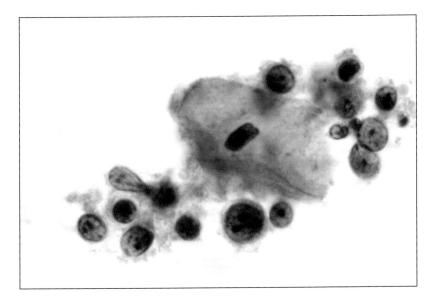

Figure 4.48

Follicular cervicitis

This field shows a mixed population of lymphoid cells surrounding an intermediate cell. Lymphocytes on their own cannot be reported as follicular cervicitis without the presence of tingible body macrophages. Lymphoma should always be borne in mind although it is very rare. (Pap HP ThinPrep®)

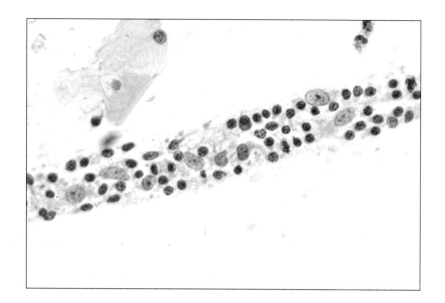

Figure 4.49

Follicular cervicitis

The appearance in conventional smears differs from those of liquid-based preparations in that the lymphoid cells are seen in large streaks as demonstrated here, rather than in clumps, admixed with histiocytes. (Pap LP Conventional smear)

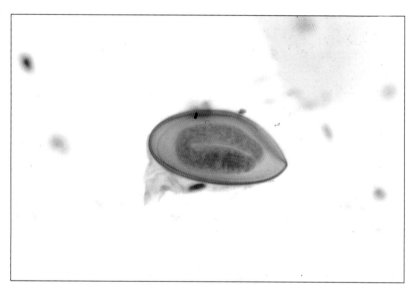

Figure 4.50

Pinworm ovum

Conventional smear showing a pinworm (*Enterobius vermicularis*) ovum with the characteristic appearance of one folded and one flattened edge. (Pap HP Conventional smear)

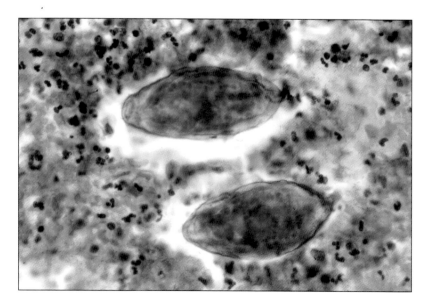

Figure 4.51

Schistosoma hematobium ova

Two *S hematobium* ova with terminal spines are seen in a blood-stained background in this conventional smear. (Pap HP Conventional smear)

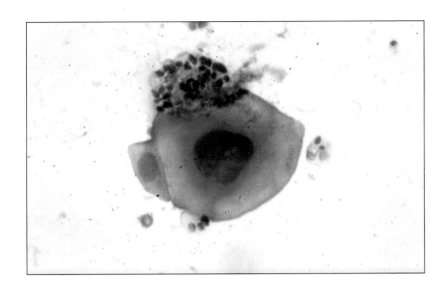

Figure 4.52

Radiation changes

This degenerating cell shows amphophilia and an enlarged but smudged nucleus—all signs of degeneration. (Pap HP Conventional smear)

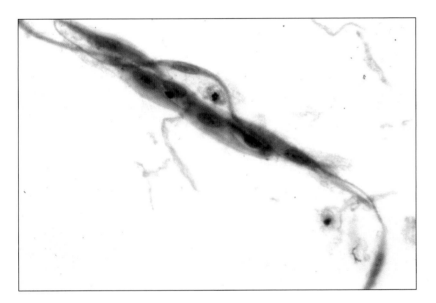

Figure 4.53

Radiation changes

Abnormal spindle cells seen in a smear following radiation treatment. (Pap HP ThinPrep®)

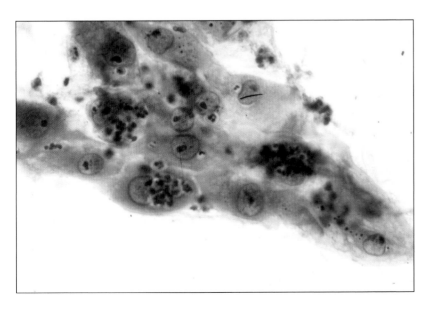

Figure 4.54

Radiation changes

This field shows a cluster of atypical epithelial cells with abundant cytoplasm, large nuclei (compared with polymorphs), prominent nucleoli, and phagocytosed polymorphs. (Pap HP ThinPrep®)

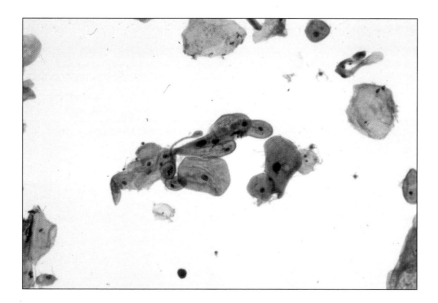

Figure 4.55

Radiation changes

There is a group of large, strangely shaped cells in the center of the field compared with the much smaller blue-staining superficial cell at 3 o'clock. (Pap LP ThinPrep®)

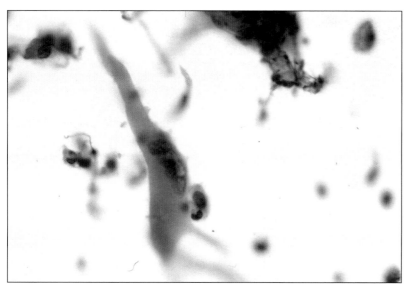

Figure 4.56

Radiation changes

A spindle-shaped cell with multiple, irregular, degenerated nuclei in a post-radiation smear. (Pap HP SurePath®)

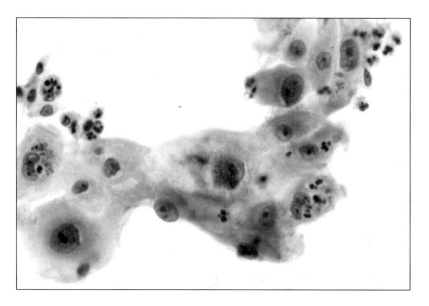

Figure 4.57

Radiation changes

These large abnormal cells with enlarged nuclei, prominent nucleoli, and phagocytosed polymorphs resemble the cells seen in the ThinPrep® smear in Figure 4.54. (Pap HP SurePath®)

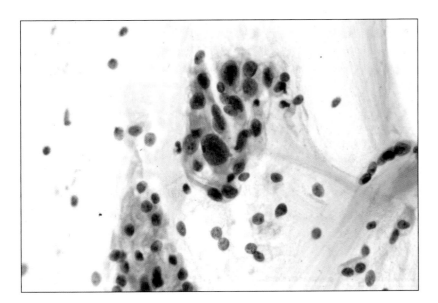

Figure 4.58

Chemotherapy effect

Conventional smear showing cells with nuclear enlargement and smudged chromatin in a patient undergoing chemotherapy. (Pap HP Conventional smear)

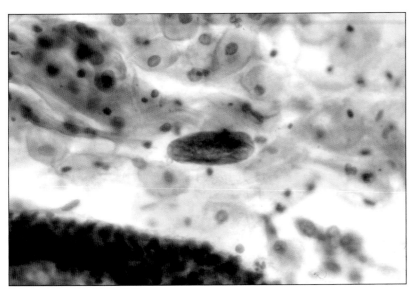

Figure 4.59

Tamoxifen effect

A large, grooved, bare nucleus is seen, surrounded by parabasal cells. No other abnormalities were seen in this conventional smear from a woman with breast cancer who was receiving tamoxifen. (Pap HP Conventional smear)

Recommended reading

1. Parashari A, Singh V, Gupta MM, et al. Significance of inflammatory cervical smears. *APMIS* 1995;**103**:273–8.

2. Eckert LO, Koutsky LA, Kiviat NB, et al. The inflammatory Papanicolaou smear: what does it mean? *Obstet Gynecol* 1995;**86**:360–6.

3. Marshall LM, Cason Z, Cabaniss DE, et al. Reactive cell change in cervicovaginal smears. *Biomed Sci Instrum* 1997;**33**:298–304.

4. Peer AK, Hoosen AA, Seedat MA, et al. Vaginal yeast infectons in diabetic women. *S Afr Med J* 1993;**83**:727–9.

5. von Maseela T. *Leptothrix vaginalis.* Morphological studies. *Fortschr Med* 1976;**94**:295–8.

6. Sardana S, Sodhani P, Agarwal SS, et al. Epidemioloic analysis of *Trichomonas vaginalis* infection in inflammatory sears. *Acta Cytol* 1994;**38**:693–7.

7. Mehta SH, Verma K. Relationship between size of *Trichomonas vaginalis* and pathogenicity. *Indian J Med Res* 1981;**74**:231–5.

8. Adad SJ, de Lima RV, Sawan ZT, et al. Frequency of *Trichomonas vaginalis, Candida* sp and *Gardnerella vaginalis* in cervical-vaginal smears in four different decades. *Sao Paolo Med J* 2001;**119**:200–5.

9. Reed BD, Huck W, Zazove P. Differentiation of *Gardnerella vaginalis, Candid albicans,* and *Trichomonas vaginalis* infections of the vagina. *J Fam Pract* 1989;**28**:673–80.

10. McLennan MT, Smith JM, McLennan CE. Diagnosis of vaginal mycosis and trichomoniasis. Reliability of cytologic smear, wet smear and culture. *Obstet Gynecol* 1972;**40**:231–4.

11. Guijon G, Paraskevas M, Rand F, et al. Vaginal microbial flora as a cofactor in the pathogenesis of uterine cervical intraepithelial neoplasia. *Int J Gynaecol Obstet* 1992;**37**:185–91.

12. Ghorab Z, Mahmood S, Schinella R. Endocervical reactive atypia: a histologic-cytologic study. *Diagn Cytopathol* 2000;**22**:342–6.

13. Ngadiman S, Yang GC. Adenomyomatous, lower uterine segment and endocervical polyps in cervicovaginal smears. *Acta Cytol* 1995;**39**:643–7.

14. Barr Soofer S, Sidawy MK. Reactive cellular change: is there an increased risk for squamous intraepithelial lesions? *Cancer* 1997;**81**:144–7.

15. Ng WK, Li AS, Cheung LK. Significance of atypical repair in liquid-based gynecologic cytology: a follow-up study with molecular analysis for human papillomavirus. *Cancer* 2003;**25**:141–8.

16. Ahmad MM. IUDs and actinomyces. *IPPF Med Bull* 1987;**21**:3–4.

17. Stowell SB, Wiley CM, Powers CN. Herpesvirus mimics. A potential pitfall in endocervical brush specimens. *Acta Cytol* 1994;**38**:43–50.

18. Rimdusit PK Yoosook C, Srivanboon S, et al. Prevalence of genital herpes simplex infection and abnormal vaginal cytology in late pregnancy in asymptomatic patients. *Int J Gynaecol Obstet* 1989;**30**:231–6.

19. Werness BA. Cytopathology of sexually transmitted disease. *Clin Lab Med* 1989;**9**:559–72.

20. Abadi MA, Barakat RR, Saigo PE. Effects of tamoxifen on cervicovaginal smears from patients with breast cancer. *Acta Cytol* 2000;**44**:141–6.

21. Yang YJ, Trapkin LK, Demoski RK, et al. The small blue cell dilemma associated with tamoxifen therapy. *Arch Pathol Lab Med* 2001;**125**:1047–50.

22. Opjorden SL, Caudill JL, Humphrey SK, Salamao DR. Small cells in cervical-vaginal smears of patients treated with tamoxifen. *Cancer* 2001;**25**:23–8.

23. Chen P, Yang CC, Chen YJ, Wang PH. Tamoxifen-induced endometrial cancer. *Eur J Gynaecol Oncol* 2003;**24**:135–7.

24. Love RR, Kurtycz DF, Dumesic Da, et al. The effects of tamoxifen on the vaginal epithelium in post-menopausal women. *J Womens Health Gend Based Med* 2000;**9**:559–63.

25. Boccardo F, Bruzzi P, Rubagotti A, et al. Estrogen-like action of tamoxifen on vaginal epithelium in breast cancer patients. *Oncology* 1981;**38**:281–5.

26. Eells TP, Alpern HD, Grzywacz C, et al. The effect of tamoxifen on cervical squamous maturation in Papanicolaou stained cervical smears of post-menopausal women. *Cytopathology* 1990;**1**:263–8.

27. Shield PW, Daunter B, Wright RG. Post-irradiation cytology of cervical cancer patients. *Cytopathology* 1992;**3**:167–82.

28. Wright JD, Herzog RJ, Mutch DG, et al. Liquid-based cytology for the postirradiation surveillance of women with gynecologic malignancies. *Gynecol Oncol* 2003;**91**:134–8.

29. Shield PW, Wright RG, Free K, Daunter B. The accuracy of cervicovaginal cytology in the detecton of recurrent cervical carcinoma following radiotherapy. *Gynecol Oncol* 1991;**41**:223–9.

30. Whitaker SJ, Blake PR, Trott PA. The value of cervical cytology in detecting recurrent squamous carcinoma of the cervix postradiotherapy. *Clin Oncol (R Coll Radiol)* 1990;**2**:254–9.

31. Shield PW. Chronic radiation effects: a orrelative study of smears and biopsies from the cervix and vagina. *Diagn Cytopathol* 1995;**13**:107–19.

32. Shield PW, Daunter B, Wright RG. Post-irradiation cytology of cervical cancer patients. *Cytopathology* 1992;**3**:167–82.

33. Frierson HF Jr, Covell JL, Andersen WA. Radiation changes in endocervical cells in brush specimens. *Diagn Cytopathol* 1990;**6**:243–7.

34. Gupta S, Gupta YN, Sanyal B. Radiation changes in vaginal and cervical cytology in carcinoma of the cervic uteri. *J Surg Oncol* 1982;**19**:71–3.

5 Squamous cell abnormalities: atypical squamous cells and low grade squamous intraepithelial lesion (LSIL)

Atypical squamous cells/ borderline changes

This category includes both atypical squamous cells of uncertain significance (ASC-US) and atypical squamous cells – cannot exclude HSIL (ASC-H) (Table 5.1).

Atypical squamous cells of undetermined significance (ASC-US)

The features that describe cells in the category of atypical squamous cells of undetermined significance include nuclear enlargement of 2.5–3 times the size of an intermediate cell nucleus, smooth nuclear outlines, and hyperchromatic, but usually evenly dispersed chromatin. The atypia does not fulfil the criteria for low grade squamous epithelial lesion (LSIL), but is worse than that seen in inflammatory/reactive changes. The UK classification for abnormal smears uses the term 'borderline' rather than ASC-US and also includes human papillomavirus (HPV) changes under the category 'borderline', not under mild dysplasia/ cervical intraepithelial neoplasia (CIN1).

Atypical squamous cells – cannot exclude high grade squamous intraepithelial lesion (ASC-H)

This category is used when small atypical cells with a high nuclear/cytoplasmic ratio, hyperchromasia and variably irregular nuclear margins are present in the smear. Because of their small size it can be difficult to determine whether these cells represent a benign condition such as immature squamous metaplasia, or are high grade dysplastic cells. The category is useful as it conveys the cytopathologist's concern to the gynecologists, and the management is the same as that for a high grade lesion (HSIL).

Table 5.1
Squamous cell abnormalities (Bethesda 2001[2])

Atypical squamous cells
- of undetermined significance (ASC-US)
- cannot exclude HSIL (ASC-H)

Low grade squamous intraepithelial lesion (LSIL/mild dysplasia/HPV)

High grade squamous intraepithelial lesion (HSIL/moderate and severe dysplasia)

Squamous cell carcinoma

Low grade squamous intraepithelial lesion/mild dysplasia/human papillomavirus changes

Both mild dysplasia and HPV changes are included in this category, and the morphologic features of both are often seen in the same smear. Typically, dysplastic cells exhibit nuclear enlargement and irregularity, abnormal chromatin, either hypo- or hyperchromatic, and no visible nucleoli. Dysplasia is graded according to the maturity of the cell; therefore, mildly dysplastic cells are the size of superficial or intermediate cells, while high grade squamous intraepithelial lesional (HSIL) cells are smaller.

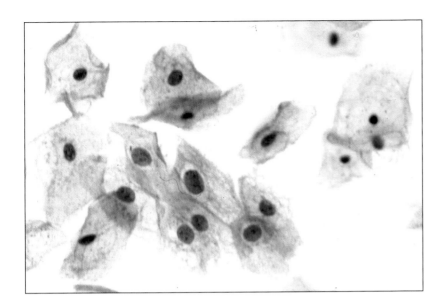

Figure 5.1

ASC-US

Some of the intermediate cells in this field show nuclear enlargement approximately 2–3 times the size of the intermediate cell nucleus at 3 o'clock. The chromatin is uniform and the nuclear margins are smooth. These features fit the definition of ASC-US. (Pap LP ThinPrep®)

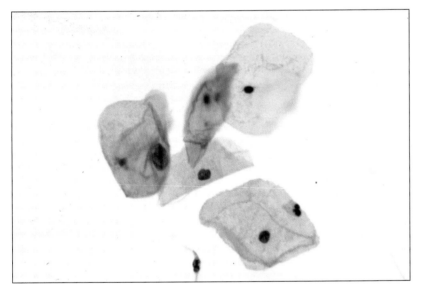

Figure 5.2

ASC-US

The cell at 9 o'clock has a nuclear size about 3 times that of the intermediate cell at 5 o'clock. The cytoplasm appears to be folded and the nucleus is hyperchromatic. (Pap HP ThinPrep®)

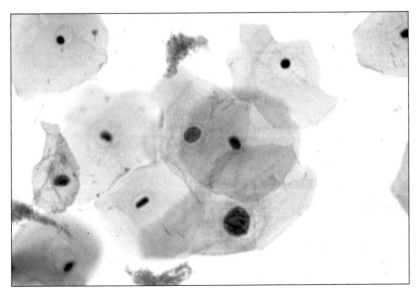

Figure 5.3

ASC-US

The cell at 6 o'clock has a nucleus at least three times the size of the intermediate cell in the center of the field but the chromatin does not support a diagnosis of anything worse than ASC-US. (Pap HP ThinPrep®)

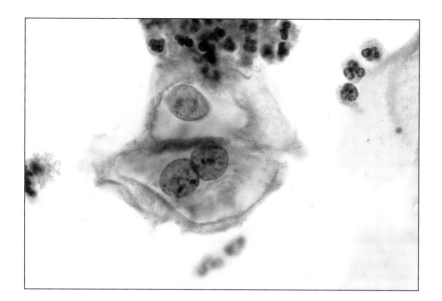

Figure 5.4

ASC-US

Note the nuclear enlargement and hint of large perinuclear haloes within these two cells. The changes are insufficient for LSIL on these two cells alone, therefore this is categorized as ASC-US. (Pap LP SurePath®)

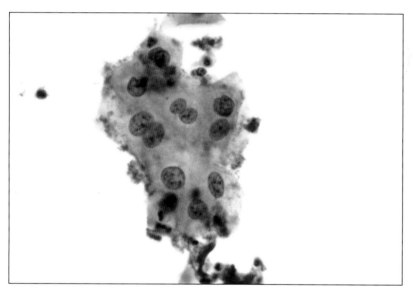

Figure 5.5

ASC-US

A group of intermediate cells showing nuclear enlargement, binucleation, and hyperchromasia. (Pap HP ThinPrep®)

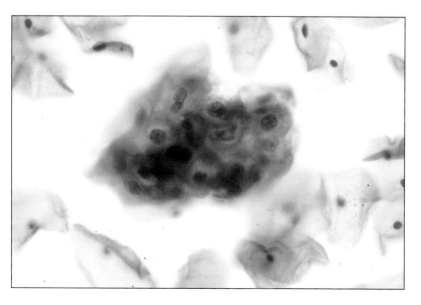

Figure 5.6

ASC-US

This cluster of degenerating cells shows pyknotic nuclei and some nuclear enlargement. Dysplasia cannot be excluded, therefore this is categorized as ASC-US. (Pap HP SurePath®)

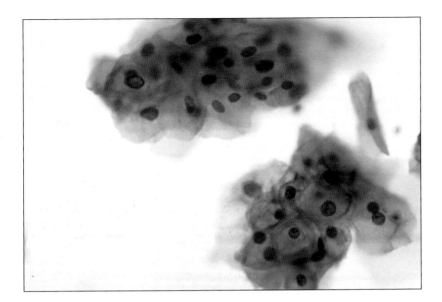

Figure 5.7

ASC-US Atypical parakeratosis

Two clusters of keratinized cells with enlarged nuclei showing evidence of degeneration are seen in this SurePath® preparation. The cells show slight nuclear enlargement compared with the folded benign cell at 3 o'clock. A binucleate cell is seen. The nuclei in the cluster above show signs of degeneration in the form of smudged, dark chromatin. These changes qualify for ASC-US but not for LSIL. (Pap HP SurePath®)

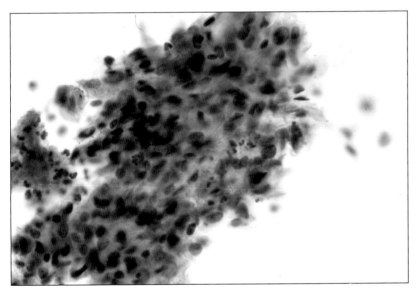

Figure 5.8

ASC-US Atypical parakeratosis

This thick cluster of small abnormal keratinized cells shows nuclear enlargement and hyperchromasia, accompanied by degenerative changes. (Pap HP ThinPrep®)

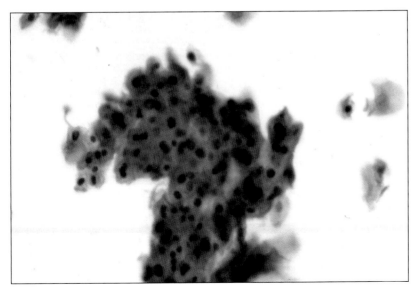

Figure 5.9

ASC-US Atypical parakeratosis

A cluster of small keratinized cells showing variable nuclear enlargement is seen here. Underlying dysplasia or HPV change cannot be excluded. (Pap HP ThinPrep®)

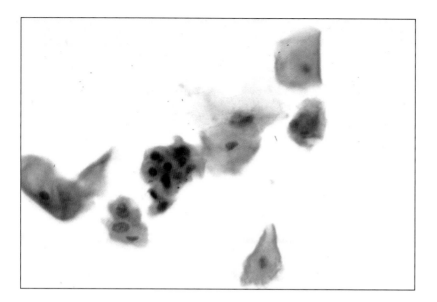

Figure 5.10

ASC-US Atypical parakeratosis

Small keratinized cells with degenerating dark nuclei, some slightly enlarged, are seen here, surrounded by mature squamous cells. (Pap HP ThinPrep®)

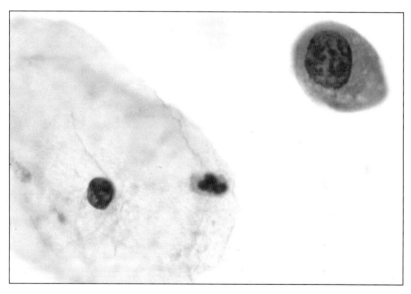

Figure 5.11

ASC-H

Next to the cyanophilic superficial cell is a small cell, smaller than a parabasal cell, with an enlarged, hyperchromatic nucleus and smooth nuclear margin. It does not quite fulfil the criteria for HSIL; it therefore is placed in the ASC-H category. Further investigation may show that this represents immature squamous metaplasia, but it could also denote a high grade lesion. (Pap HP ThinPrep®)

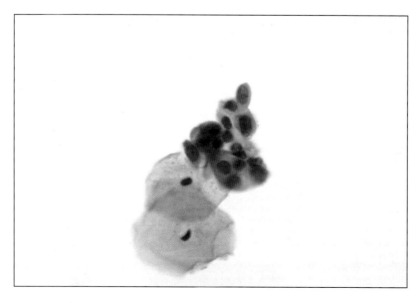

Figure 5.12

ASC-H

Note the cluster of small cells that are approximately the size of parabasal cells, with high nuclear : cytoplasmic ratios, hyperchromasia, and variable sizes, adjacent to two superficial cells. These most likely represent immature/atypical squamous metaplasia but HSIL cannot be excluded, therefore this is categorized as ASC-H. (Pap LP ThinPrep®)

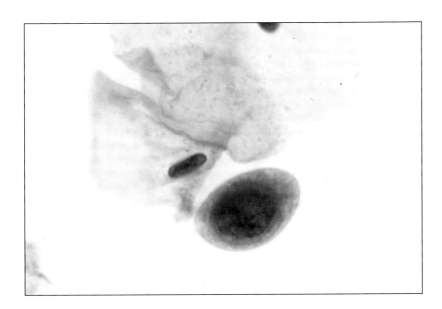

Figure 5.13

ASC-H

The small cell near the intermediate cells shows a high nuclear : cytoplasmic ratio, hyperchromasia, and sharply defined cytoplasm, probably representing immature squamous metaplasia but HSIL cannot be ruled out, so this is characterized as ASC-H. (Pap HP ThinPrep®)

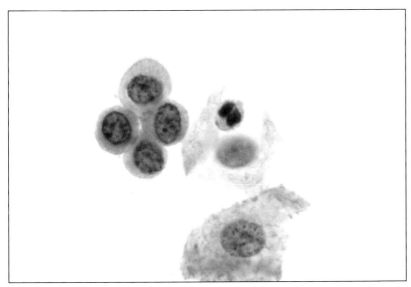

Figure 5.14

ASC-H

The group of four small cells with a high nuclear : cytoplasmic ratio and hyperchromatic nuclei are suggestive of, but do not have all the criteria of HSIL and therefore are placed in the ASC-H category. Clinical management of this group is the same as for HSIL. (Pap HP ThinPrep®)

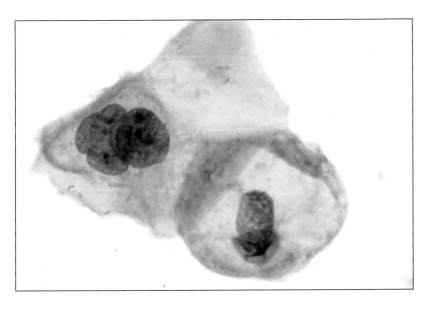

Figure 5.15

LSIL/mild dysplasia

Two mildly dysplastic cells with enlarged, irregular, hyperchromatic nuclei are seen here. One cell is multinucleated while the other shows indistinct features of HPV change. (Pap OI ThinPrep®)

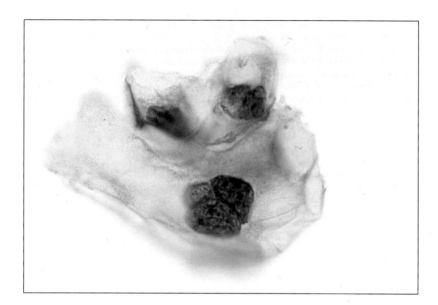

Figure 5.16

LSIL/mild dysplasia

Mildly dysplastic cells in a SurePath® smear, showing multinucleation. (Pap HP SurePath®)

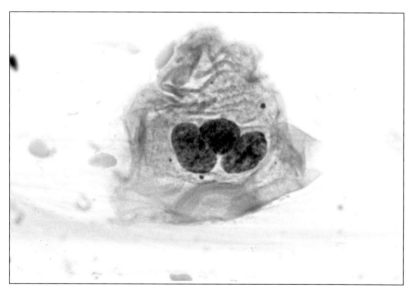

Figure 5.17

LSIL/mild dysplasia

A mildly dysplastic cell in a conventional smear, showing multinucleation. (Pap HP Conventional smear)

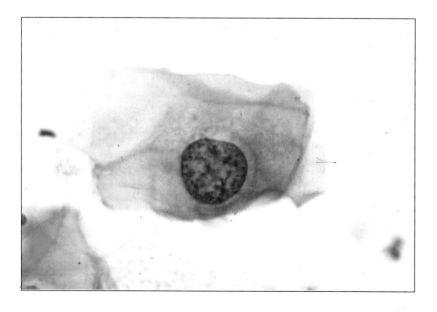

Figure 5.18

LSIL/mild dysplasia

A mildly dysplastic cell is seen with an enlarged nucleus and irregularly distributed clumped chromatin, which is obviously abnormal. (Pap HP ThinPrep®)

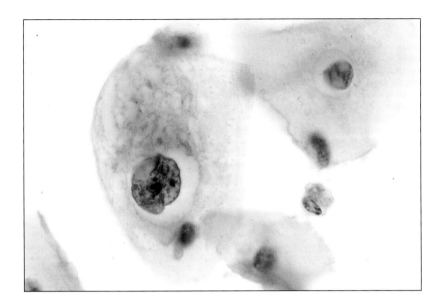

Figure 5.19

LSIL/mild dysplasia

This abnormal cell shows the features of mild dysplasia. It is large with an enlarged, hyperchromatic nucleus, an irregular nuclear margin and irregularly clumped chromatin. Note that the edge of the nucleus is folded over in one area. (Pap HP ThinPrep®)

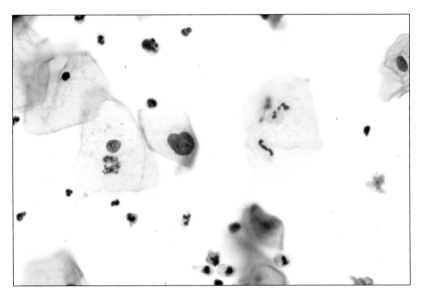

Figure 5.20

LSIL/mild dysplasia

The cell in the center shows features of mild dysplasia with an enlarged hyperchromatic nucleus. (Pap HP SurePath®)

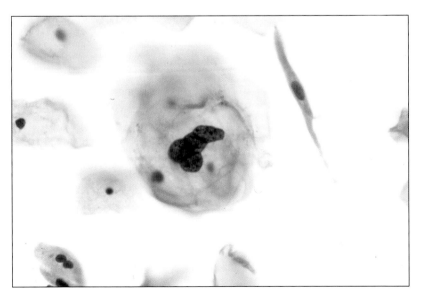

Figure 5.21

LSIL/mild dysplasia

A mildly dysplastic cell with an abnormal hyperchromatic, multinucleated nucleus. (Pap HP SurePath®)

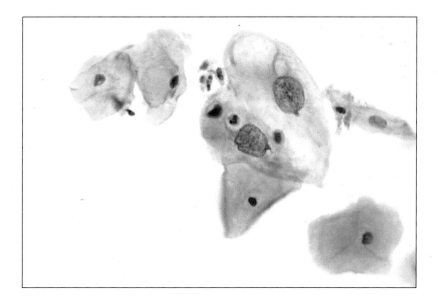

Figure 5.22

LSIL/mild dysplasia

The mildly dysplastic heart-shaped cell in this field has two irregular nuclei with pale abnormal chromatin. Hypochromatic nuclei are not an indicator of degeneration as degenerated nuclei are hyperchromatic with 'smudged' or pyknotic chromatin. Pale nuclei have an abundance of euchromatin (active chromatin) (Pap HP ThinPrep®)

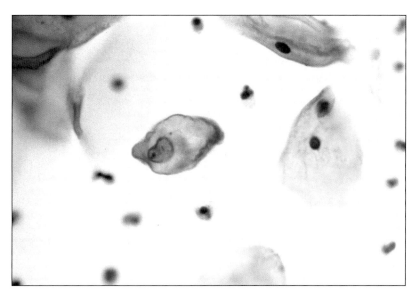

Figure 5.23

LSIL/mild dysplasia

This is a SurePath® smear showing a mildly dysplastic cell with pale chromatin. (Pap HP SurePath®)

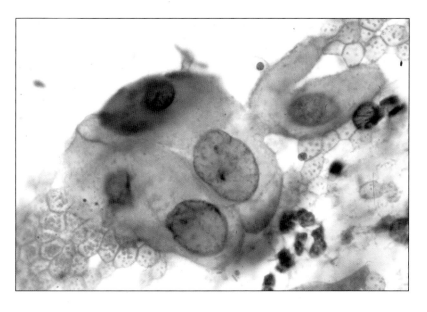

Figure 5.24

LSIL/mild dysplasia

A group of mildly dysplastic cells with large nuclei and pale but abnormal chromatin. Pale dysplastic cells are seen in conventional as well as liquid-based smears but are easiest to detect in ThinPrep® preparations. (Pap OI Conventional smear)

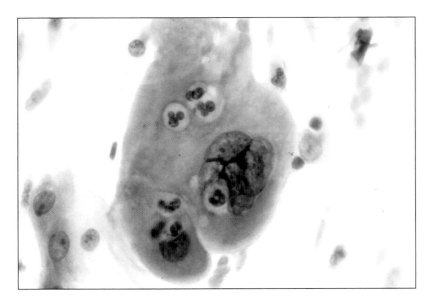

Figure 5.25

LSIL/mild dysplasia

This mildly dysplastic cell has engulfed neutrophils. Phagocytosis of inflammatory cells and other dysplastic cells is not uncommon in dysplasia. (Pap HP Conventional smear)

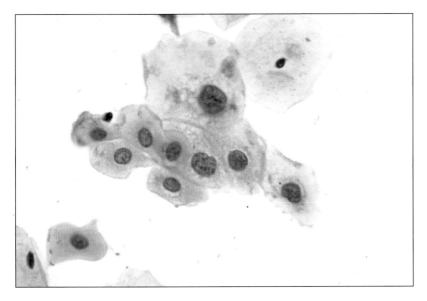

Figure 5.26

LSIL/mild dysplasia

A sheet composed of mildly dysplastic cells is seen with an adjacent superficial cell. (Pap HP ThinPrep®)

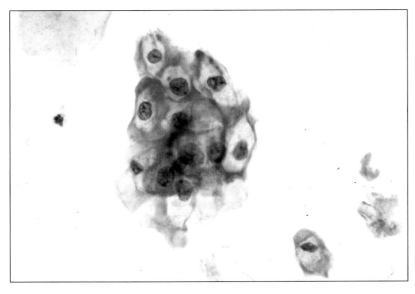

Figure 5.27

LSIL/mild dysplasia/HPV

This cluster of mildly dysplastic cells shows nuclear enlargement and abnormal chromatin as well as a halo and an irregularly thickened cytoplasmic rim indicative of HPV changes. (Pap HP ThinPrep®)

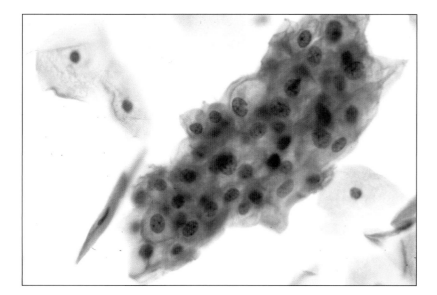

Figure 5.28

LSIL/mild dysplasia

The cluster of cells seen here shows mildly dysplastic changes with nuclei 3–4 times the size of an intermediate cell nucleus and abnormal chromatin. Some cells have haloes suggesting HPV changes.
(Pap HP SurePath®)

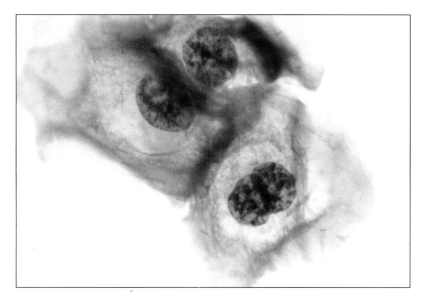

Figure 5.29

LSIL/HPV changes

This high power view of koilocytes with mild dysplasia shows abnormal nuclei with binucleation, chromatin clumping and clearing, haloes and irregularly thickened cytoplasmic edges. (Pap OI ThinPrep®)

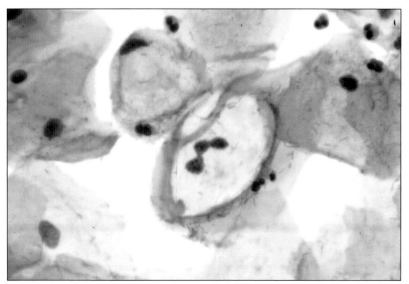

Figure 5.30

LSIL/HPV changes (borderline changes)

The cell in the center of the field is a koilocyte, with three small pyknotic nuclei, a well-defined halo and thickened cytoplasmic edge. The adjacent cyanophilic cell is glycogenated and is not a koilocyte. (Pap LP SurePath®)

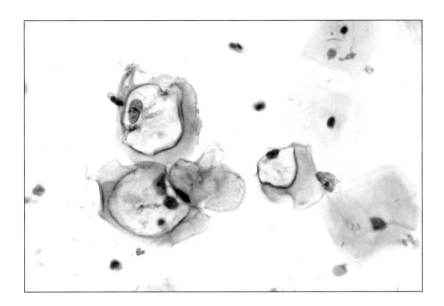

Figure 5.31

LSIL/HPV changes (borderline changes)

This is a ThinPrep® Pap smear from a premenopausal woman (note the benign superficial cells in the background). It shows the three characteristic features of koilocytes: unevenly thickened cytoplasmic rims, an abnormal nucleus (binucleation in one cell), and sharply defined cytoplasmic haloes. (Pap LP ThinPrep®)

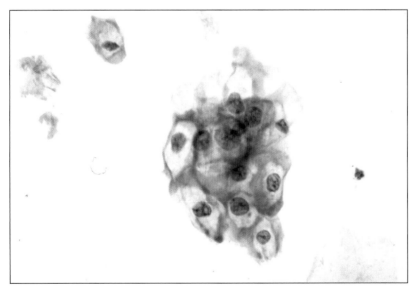

Figure 5.32

LSIL/HPV changes (borderline changes)

This is a cluster of koilocytes in a background of cytolysis. Excessive cytolysis can sometimes make grading of dysplasia difficult. (Pap HP ThinPrep®)

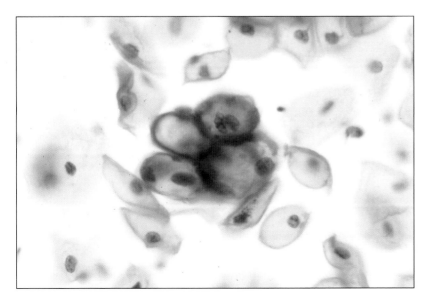

Figure 5.33

LSIL/HPV changes (borderline changes)

This preparation shows cells at various planes in the field. The cells in the center are koilocytes with hyperchromatic nuclei, thickened rims, and haloes that are not sharply defined. Parabasal and intermediate cells are seen in the background. (Pap LP SurePath®)

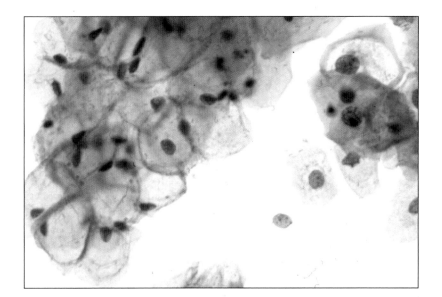

Figure 5.34

LSIL/HPV changes (borderline changes)

In this field there is a koilocyte at the upper right, while on the left is a cluster of navicular cells with thickened edges and clear cytoplasm, which can sometimes mimic HPV changes. (Pap HP ThinPrep®)

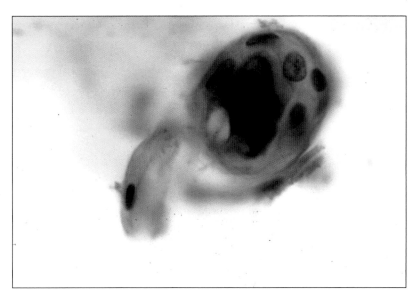

Figure 5.35

Dysplastic pearl

This epithelial pearl is composed of cells with enlarged hyperchromatic nuclei. Dysplastic cells were seen in other fields of this smear. (Pap HP SurePath®: dysk pearl SP)

Recommended reading

1. ChangChien CC, Lin H, Eng HL, et al. Clinical implication of atypical squamous cells of undetermined significance with or without favoring high-grade squamous intraepithelial lesion on cervical smears. *Changgeng Yi Xue Za Zhi* 1999;**22**:579–85.

2. Solomon D, Davey D, Kurman R, et al. The 2001 Bethesda System: terminology for reporting results of cervical cytology. *JAMA* 2002;**287**:2114–9.

3. Selvaggi SM. Reporting of atypical squamous cells, cannot exclude a high-grade squamous intraepithelial lesion (ASC-H) on cervical samples: is it significant? *Diagn Cytopathol* 2003;**29**:38–41.

4. Guerrini L, Sama D, Visani M, et al. Is it possible to define a better ASCUS class in cervicovaginal screening? A review of 187 cases. *Acta Cytol* 2001;**45**:532–6.

5. Acs G, Gupta PK, Baloch ZW. Glandular and squamous atypia and intraepithelial lesions in atrophic cervicovaginal smears. One institution's experience. *Acta Cytol* 2000;**44**:611–17.

6. Vlahos NP, Dragisic KG, Wallach EE, et al. Clinical significance of the qualification of atypical squamous cells of undetermined significance: An analysis on the basis of histologic diagnoses. *Am J Obstet Gynecol* 2000;**182**:885–90.

7. Genest DR. Dean B, Lee K, et al. Qualifying the cytologic diagosis of 'atypical squamous cells of undetermined significance' affects the predictive value of a squamous intraepithelial lesion on subsequent biopsy. *Arch Pathol Lab Med* 1998;**122**:338–41.

8. Pitman MB, Cibas ES, Powers CN, et al. Reducing or eliminating use of the category of atypical squamous cells of undetermined significance decreases the diagnostic accuracy of the Papanicolaou smear. *Cancer* 2002;**96**:128–34.

9. ASCUS-LSIL Triage Study (ALTS) Group. Results of a randomized trial on the management of cytology interpretations of atypical squamous cells of undetermined significance. *Am J Obstet Gynecol* 2003;**188**:1383–92.

10. Abramovich CM, Wasman JK, Siekkinen P, Abdul-Karim FW. Histopathologic correlation of atypical parakeratosis diagnosed cervicovaginal cytology. *Acta Cytol* 2003;**47**:405–9.

11. Yang M, Zachariah S. ASCUS cervical cytologic smears. Clinical significance. *J Reprod Med* 1997;**42**:329–31.

12. Arbyn M, Buntinx F, Van Ranst M, et al. Virologic versus cytologic triage of women with equivocal Pap smears: a meta-analysis of the accuracy to detect high-grade intraepithelial neoplasia. *J Natl Cancer Inst* 2004;**96**:280–93.

13. Crabtree D, Unkraut A, Cozens D, et al. Role for HPV testing in ASCUS: a cytologic-histologic correlation. *Diagn Cytopathol* 2002;**27**:382–6.

14. Hong IS, Marshalleck J, Williams RH, et al. Comparative analysis of a liquid-based Pap test and concurrent HPV DNA assay of residual samples. A study of 608 cases. *Acta Cytol* 2002;**46**:828–34.

15. Coach S, Cason Z, Benghuzzi H. An evaluation of infectious diseases in cervicovaginal smears from patients with atypical cells of undetermined significance. *Biomed Sci Instrum* 2001;**37**:167–72.

16. Malik SN, Wilkinson EJ, Drew PA, et al. Do qualifiers of ASCUS distinguish between low- and high-risk patients? *Acta Cytol* 1999;**43**:376–80.

17. Sherman ME, Solomon D, Schiffman M, ASCUS LSIL Triage Study Group. Qualification of ASCUS. A comparison of equivocal LSIL and equivocal HSIL cervical cytology in the ASCUS LSIL Triage Study. *Am J Clin Pathol* 2001;**116**:386–94.

18. Williams ML, Rimm DL, Pedigo MA, Frable WJ. Atypical squamous cells of undetermined significance: correlative histologic and follow-up studies from an academic medical center. *Diagn Cytopathol* 1997;**16**:1–7.

19. Cengel KA, Day SJ, Davis-Devine S, et al. Effectiveness of the SurePath liquid-based Pap test in automated screening and in detection of HSIL. *Diagn Cytopathol* 2003;**29**:250–5.

20. Nasser SM, Cibas ES, Crum CP, Faquin WC. The significance of the Papanicolaou smear diagnosis of low-grade squamous intraepithelial lesion cannot exclude high-grade squamous intraepithelial lesion. *Cancer* 2003;**99**:272–6.

21. Hall S, Wu TC, Soudi N, Sherman ME. Low-grade squamous intraepithelial lesions: cytologic predictor of biopsy confirmation. *Diagn Cytopathol* 1994;**10**:3–9.

22. Schiffman M, Solomon D. Findings to date from the ASCUS-LSIL Triage Study (ALTS). *Arch Pathol Lab Med* 2003;**127**:946–9.

23. ASCUS-LSIL Triage Study (ALTS) Group. A randomized trial on the management of low-grade squamous intraepithelial cytology interpretations. *Am J Obstet Gynecol* 2003;**188**:1393–400.

24. Oh YL, Shin KJ, Han J, Kim DS. Significance of high-risk human papillomavirus detection by polymerase chain reaction in primary cervical cancer screening. *Cytopathology* 2001;**12**:75–83.

25. McGrath CM, Kurtis JD, Yu GH. Evaluation of mild-to-moderate dysplasia on cervical-endocervical (Pap) smear: a subgroup of patients who bridge LSIL and HSIL. *Diagn Cytopathol* 2000;**23**:245–8.

26. Infantolino C, Fabris P, Infantolino D, et al. Usefulness of human papilloma virus testing in the screening of cervical cancer precursor lesions: a retrospective study in 314 cases. *Eur J Obstet Gynecol Reprod Biol* 2000;**93**:71–5.

6 Squamous cell abnormalities: high grade squamous intraepithelial lesion and squamous cell carcinoma

High grade squamous intraepithelial lesion

High grade squamous intraepithelial lesion (HSIL) encompasses both moderate dysplasia/cervical intraepithelial neoplasia 2 (CIN2) and severe dysplasia/cervical intraepithelial neoplasia 3 (CIN3). Moderately dysplastic cells are about the size of parabasal cells, with a high nuclear:cytoplasmic ratio, the nucleus occupying approximately two-thirds of the cell. The nuclear margin is often irregular and the chromatin is abnormal, varying from hypochromatic to hyperchromatic. The cells may be single or in clusters. Severely dysplastic cells are very small, approximately the size of basal cells (which are never seen in a Pap smear), with enlarged nuclei that occupy almost the whole cell. The cells may be single or in syncytial groups (i.e. no cytoplasmic boundaries can be identified). The chromatin is abnormally pale or hyperchromatic and the nuclear outlines vary from smooth to irregular. The cytoplasm is often delicate and wispy and may be torn off the cell, leaving abnor-mal large bare nuclei in the background. These large abnormal nuclei are most often associated with severe dysplasia and may be used as a clue to the presence of this lesion although they are not diagnostic. HSIL cells in groups can resemble reactive endocervical cells, especially when the nuclei are hypochromatic. Nucleoli are not a feature of dysplasia. Low grade squamous intra-epithelial lesion (LSIL) cells may accompany HSIL cells.

Features that are suggestive of invasion on a Pap smear containing mostly HSIL cells include pleomorphism, nucleoli, spindle, fiber, and tad-pole cells, keratinization, and tumor diathesis. Nucleoli alone without the other features suggest microinvasion.

Squamous cell carcinoma

The features of invasion include pleomorphism with large as well as small cells, cells that are round, spindle-shaped or fiber cells, and the presence of nucleoli. Tumor diathesis, which comprises proteinaceous material, neutrophil polymorphs, red blood cells, and degenerating tumor cells, is usually present. Microinvasion is often difficult to recognize in a Pap smear unless nucleoli are easily visualized. A few fiber cells in a smear do not constitute invasion; they are more likely to represent involvement of endocervical glands by severe dysplasia. Keratinized cells are often seen in squamous carcinoma, but are also a feature of large keratinizing cell severe dysplasia.

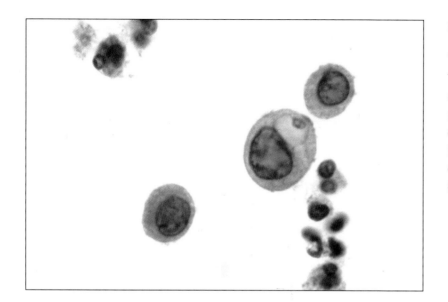

Figure 6.1

HSIL/moderate dysplasia

The three small abnormal cells in the center of the field show high nuclear:cytoplasmic ratios and abnormal chromatin. More cytoplasm is seen than in severely dysplastic cells. Compare the cell sizes with the adjacent polymorphs. (Pap OI ThinPrep®)

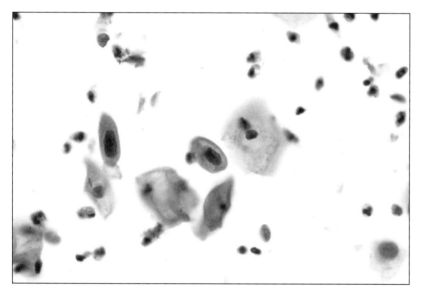

Figure 6.2

HSIL/moderate dysplasia

Two moderately dysplastic cells the size of parabasal cells are seen in the center of this field. (Pap HP SurePath®)

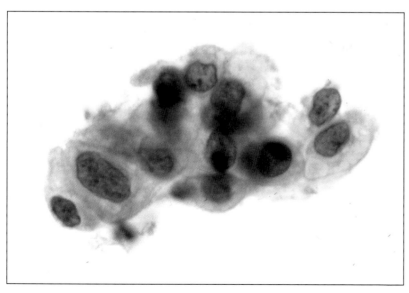

Figure 6.3

HSIL/moderate dysplasia

This is a cluster of moderately dysplastic cells with a high nuclear:cytoplasmic ratio, irregular nuclear margins and abnormal chromatin. Note the delicate cytoplasm. (Pap HP ThinPrep®)

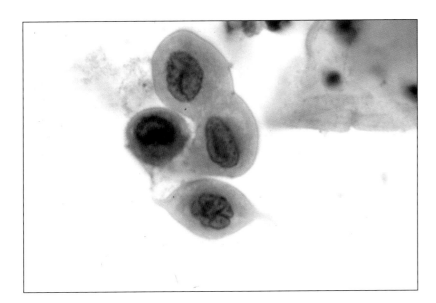

Figure 6.4

HSIL/moderate dysplasia

The small cells in the center appear metaplastic but have markedly irregular nuclear margins and abnormal chromatin, placing them in the HSIL category. (Pap HP ThinPrep®)

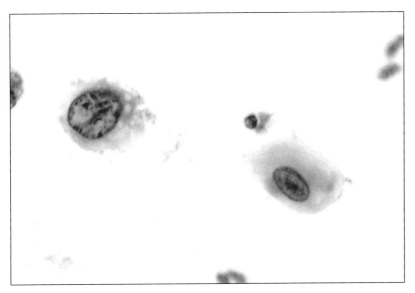

Figure 6.5

HSIL/moderate dysplasia

The cell on the left with an abnormal nucleus and delicate cytoplasm is a moderately dysplastic cell, while the one on the right with denser cytoplasm is a benign squamous metaplastic cell. (Pap HP ThinPrep®)

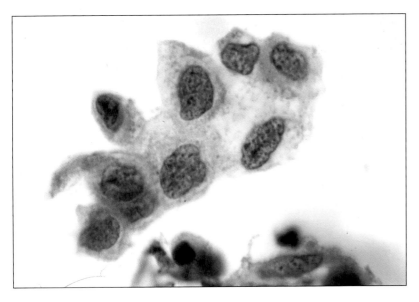

Figure 6.6

HSIL/moderate dysplasia

Group of moderately dysplastic cells with irregular hyperchromatic nuclei. (Pap HP SurePath®)

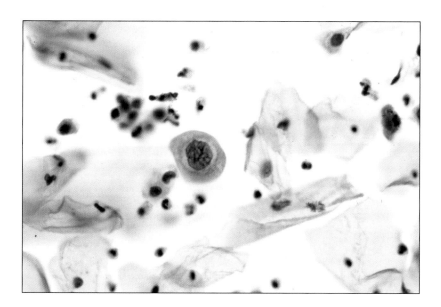

Figure 6.7

HSIL/moderate dysplasia

The moderately dysplastic cell in the center of the field is the size of a parabasal cell with an enlarged, irregular, hyperchromatic nucleus. (Pap HP SurePath®)

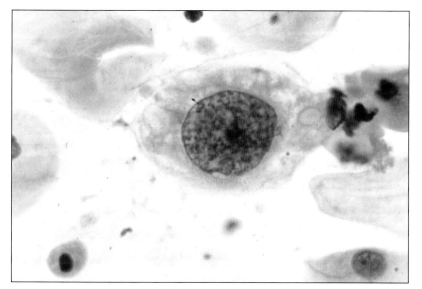

Figure 6.8

HSIL/moderate dysplasia

This is a moderately dysplastic cell with an enlarged nucleus showing abnormal clumping and clearing of chromatin, in a conventional smear. (Pap OI. Conventional smear)

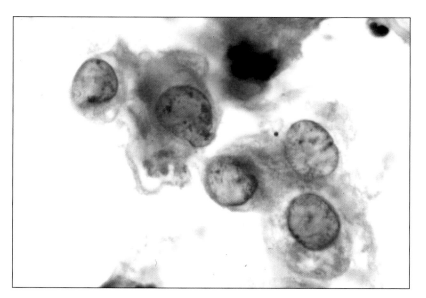

Figure 6.9

HSIL/moderate dysplasia

A cluster of moderately dysplastic cells with rounded nuclei and abnormally pale chromatin. Note the delicate cytoplasm. (Pap HP ThinPrep®)

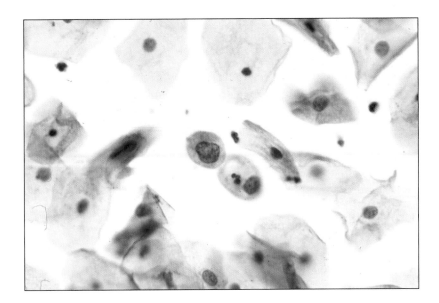

Figure 6.10

HSIL/moderate dysplasia

A SurePath® smear showing a moderately dysplastic cell with a pale, hypochromatic nucleus. The cytoplasm in these preparations is not as delicate as it is with ThinPrep®. (Pap HP SP SurePath®)

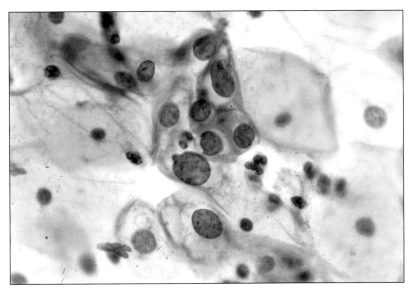

Figure 6.11

HSIL/moderate dysplasia

This is a conventional smear showing a cluster of moderately dysplastic cells with pale nuclei and delicate cytoplasm. There are also some mildly dysplastic cells in this field. (Pap HP Conventional smear)

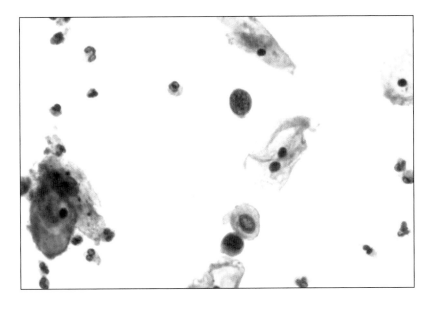

Figure 6.12

HSIL/severe dysplasia

This low power view shows scattered single small dark cells in the background of an otherwise normal appearing ThinPrep®. These are a clue to the presence of severe dysplasia and should be carefully examined under high power to avoid missing the diagnosis. (Pap LP ThinPrep®)

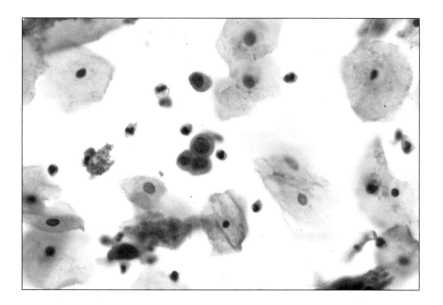

Figure 6.13

HSIL/severe dysplasia

In the center of the field there are three small hyperchromatic cells with high nuclear : cytoplasmic ratio. Similar cells are present at 12 o'clock and 7 o'clock. The appearances suggest HSIL but the cells need to be examined under higher magnification to confirm the diagnosis. (Pap LP SurePath®)

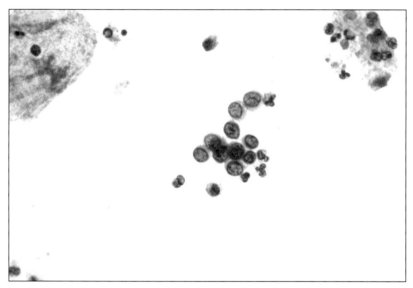

Figure 6.14

HSIL/severe dysplasia

This group of small cells shows a high nuclear : cytoplasmic ratio, smooth, round nuclei the size of polymorphs, abnormal chromatin, and minimal delicate cytoplasm. (Pap LP ThinPrep®)

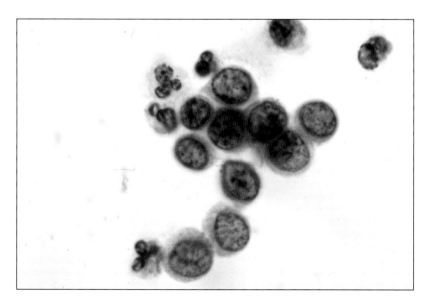

Figure 6.15

HSIL/severe dysplasia

On higher magnification these small cells show a marked clumping and clearing of chromatin and little cytoplasm, mostly delicate but denser in the cell at 12 o'clock. (Pap OI ThinPrep®)

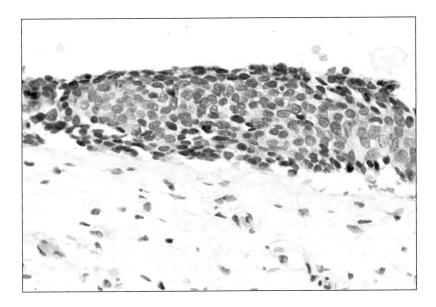

Figure 6.16

HSIL/severe dysplasia biopsy

Cervical biopsy showing that the whole thickness of the epithelium is composed of small undifferentiated hyperchromatic cells similar to those seen in the Pap smear shown in Figure 6.15. (H&E LP)

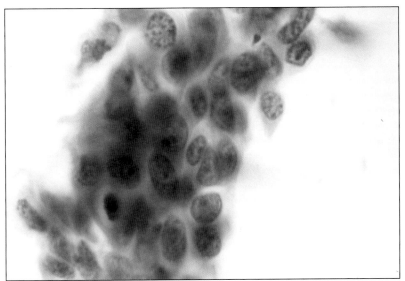

Figure 6.17

HSIL/severe dysplasia

These overlapping cells are in a tight cluster. They show a high nuclear: cytoplasmic ratio and clumping and clearing of chromatin. (Pap HP SurePath®)

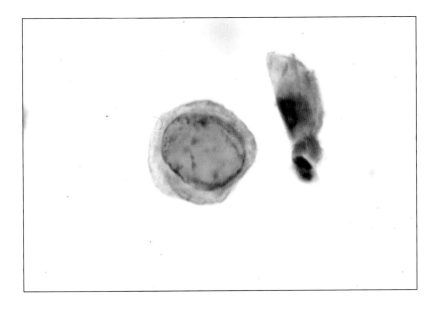

Figure 6.18

HSIL/severe dysplasia

This severely dysplastic cell has a high nuclear: cytoplasmic ratio and abnormal pale chromatin (euchromatin) with irregular strands of darkly staining heterochromatin. (Pap OI ThinPrep®)

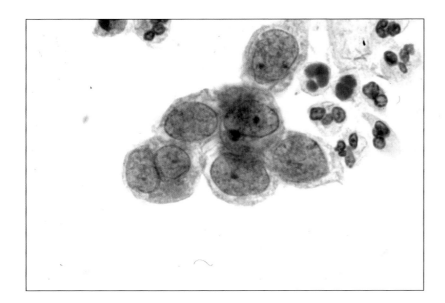

Figure 6.19

HSIL/severe dysplasia

A cluster of small cells with smooth nuclear margins, pale chromatin, and delicate cytoplasm is shown here. The presence of a nucleolus in some of the cells raises the possibility of microinvasion. (Pap OI Conventional smear)

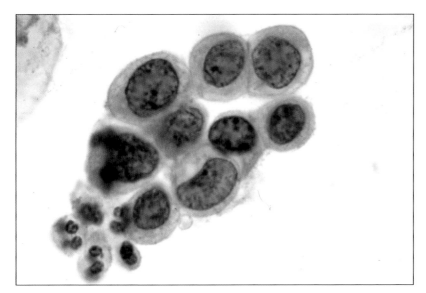

Figure 6.20

HSIL/severe dysplasia

This loose cluster of small cells has abnormal clumped and cleared chromatin and delicate cytoplasm. It is essential to note that the chromatin of dysplastic cells may be either hyper- or hypochromatic in all types of preparations: conventional smears, ThinPrep®, and SurePath® slides. (Pap OI ThinPrep®)

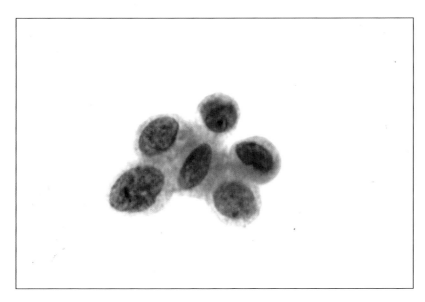

Figure 6.21

HSIL/severe dysplasia

This is a cluster of severely dysplastic cells with hyperchromatic nuclei and even less cytoplasm than the cells seen in Figure 6.20. (Pap OI ThinPrep®)

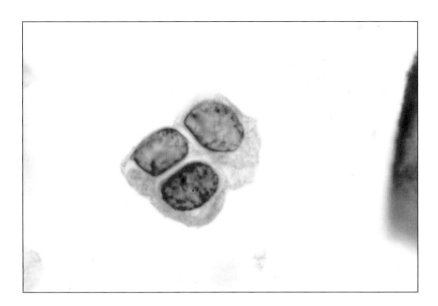

Figure 6.22

HSIL/severe dysplasia

These severely dysplastic cells display pale nuclei rather than hyperchromasia. (Pap HP SurePath®)

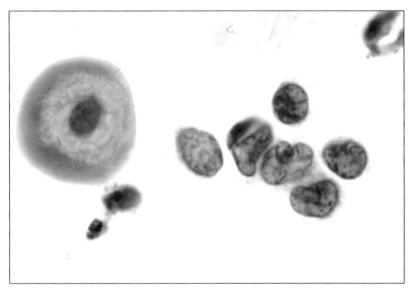

Figure 6.23

HSIL/severe dysplasia

The cells in the center of the field are much smaller than the parabasal cell on the left and display marked nuclear irregularities, irregularly cleared chromatin, and minimal cytoplasm. (Pap OI ThinPrep®)

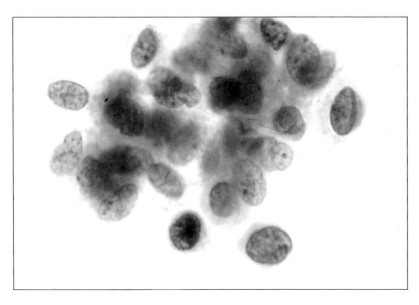

Figure 6.24

HSIL/severe dysplasia

This syncytial cluster of severely dysplastic cells may be mistaken for glandular neoplasia because of the delicate cytoplasm. The chromatin is pale but abnormal. (Pap OI ThinPrep®)

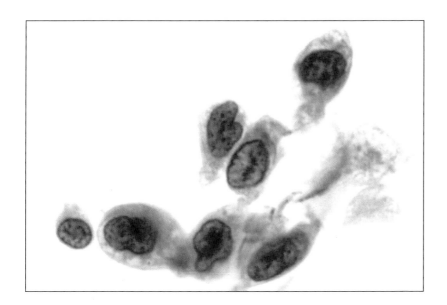

Figure 6.25

HSIL/severe dysplasia

Note the irregular nuclear margins, abnormally clumped hromatin and delicate cytoplasm of these severely dysplastic cells. (Pap OI ThinPrep®)

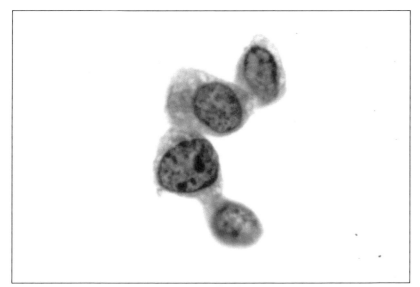

Figure 6.26

HSIL/severe dysplasia

These severely dysplastic cells display abnormally clumped chromatin and delicate, lacy cytoplasm. The cytoplasm is often stripped leaving abnormal bare nuclei. This feature is of importance in ThinPrep® smears, but not in SurePath® as bare nuclei are found in all types of smear in the latter. (Pap HP ThinPrep®)

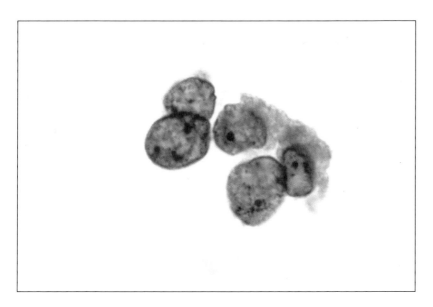

Figure 6.27

HSIL/severe dysplasia bare nuclei

This cluster is composed mainly of large bare nuclei with the features of dysplasia and a few cells with cytoplasm. While they are not diagnostic, bare nuclei should be regarded as clues to the presence of severe dysplasia. (Pap OI ThinPrep®)

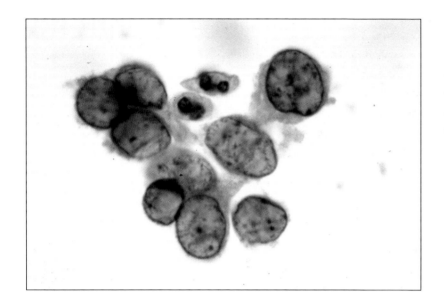

Figure 6.28

HSIL/severe dysplasia bare nuclei

Some of the severely dysplastic cells in this group have a small amount of cytoplasm, while others are bare nuclei with the same abnormal pale chromatin pattern. (Pap OI TP)

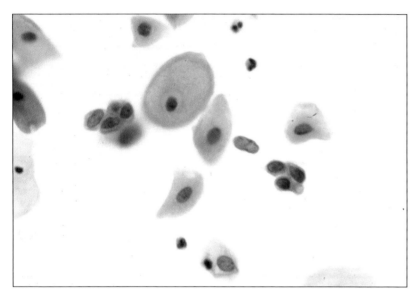

Figure 6.29

HSIL/severe dysplasia in atrophy

Small clusters of small severely dysplastic cells with irregular nuclei are seen among the parabasal cells. Note the large bare nucleus although this cannot be used as a clue in SurePath® preparations as even benign smears can show this feature. (Pap HP SurePath®)

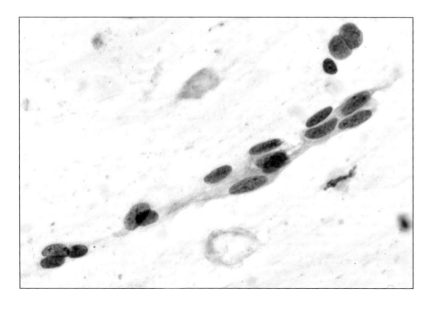

Figure 6.30

HSIL/severe dysplasia

The spindle-shaped cells seen in this atrophic smear were suspicious for HSIL as the chromatin was too coarse for parabasal cells; also there are abnormal bare nuclei. This would be reported as ASC-H using Bethesda 2001 criteria. See the biopsy image in Figure 6.31. (Pap HP Conventional smear)

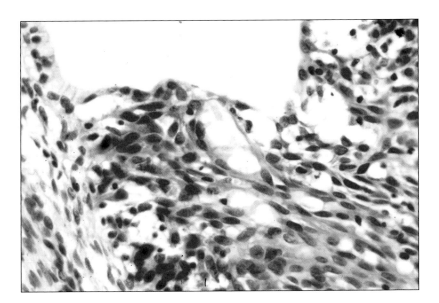

Figure 6.31

HSIL/severe dysplasia

This biopsy of the case illustrated in Figure 6.30 shows involvement of an endocervical gland by spindle-shaped severely dysplastic cells. (H&E HP)

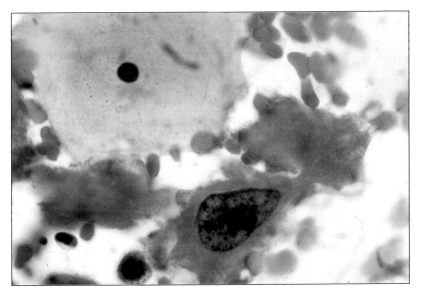

Figure 6.32

HSIL/keratinizing severe dysplasia

Note the keratinized severely dysplastic cell adjacent to a superficial cell. (Pap HP Conventional smear)

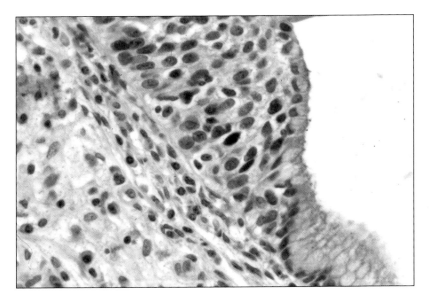

Figure 6.33

CIN3 involving glands

This biopsy shows severely dysplastic cells within an endocervical gland. Note that some of the nuclei are becoming spindle-shaped. See Pap smear appearance in Figure 6.34. (H&E HP)

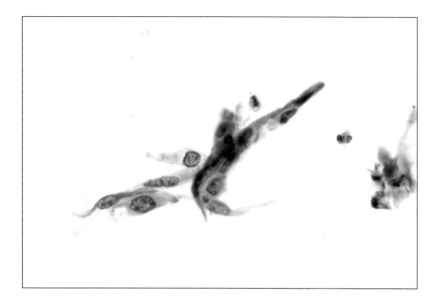

Figure 6.34

CIN3 involving glands

When rare small groups of atypical fiber cells are seen accompanying severely dysplastic cells, they are often indicative of gland involvement by CIN3 rather than invasive carcinoma. Rarely, severely dysplastic cells are seen in a sheet, continuous with benign endocervical cells, denoting gland involvement. See Figure 6.41 for comparison. (Pap HP ThinPrep®)

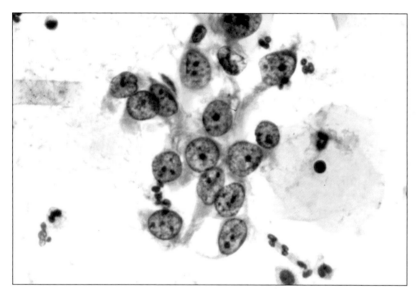

Figure 6.35

HSIL/microinvasion

This loose cluster of severely dysplastic cells shows prominent nucleoli suggestive of microinvasion. (Pap HP ThinPrep®)

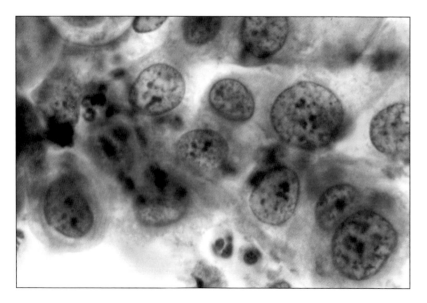

Figure 6.36

HSIL/microinvasion

The cells in this cluster show abnormally clumped, unevenly distributed chromatin, and smooth nuclear margins. The presence of nucleoli in these severely dysplastic cells is suggestive of microinvasion. (Pap OI Conventional smear)

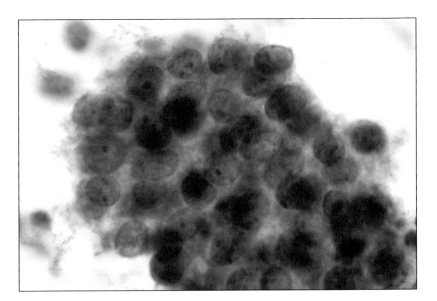

Figure 6.37

HSIL/microinvasion

This syncytial group of cells shows overlapping round nuclei, abnormal chromatin, and delicate cytoplasm. Some cells contain large nucleoli. These are severely dysplastic cells showing features suggestive of microinvasion. (Pap HP ThinPrep®)

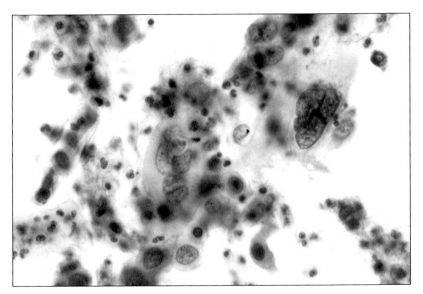

Figure 6.38

Squamous cell carcinoma

Large pleomorphic squamous carcinoma cells are seen in a 'dirty' background containing degenerating neutrophil polymorphs. (Pap HP ThinPrep®)

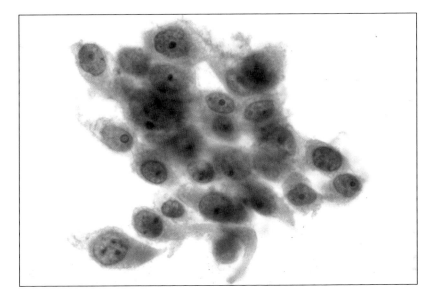

Figure 6.39

Squamous cell carcinoma

A loose cluster of severely dysplastic cells with prominent nucleoli, granular chromatin, and irregular nuclear margins is seen in this ThinPrep® smear. Nucleoli in dysplastic cells are evidence of an invasive tumor. (Pap OI ThinPrep®)

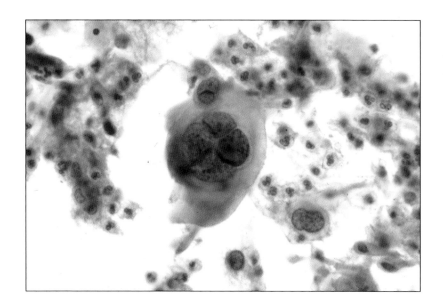

Figure 6.40

Squamous cell carcinoma

This ThinPrep® smear shows an extremely large pleomorphic tumor cell surrounded by much smaller carcinoma cells and polymorphs. (Pap HP ThinPrep®)

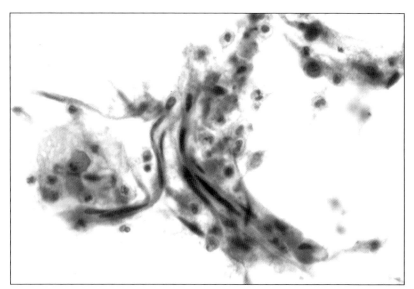

Figure 6.41

Squamous cell carcinoma

Fiber cells are a common feature of invasive squamous carcinoma. These fiber cells are accompanied by more rounded squamous carcinoma cells. See Figure 6.34 for comparison with CIN3 involving glands. (Pap HP ThinPrep®)

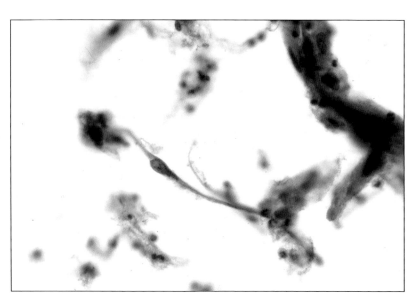

Figure 6.42

Squamous cell carcinoma

Spindle-shaped cells may be seen in squamous carcinomas. (Pap HP ThinPrep®)

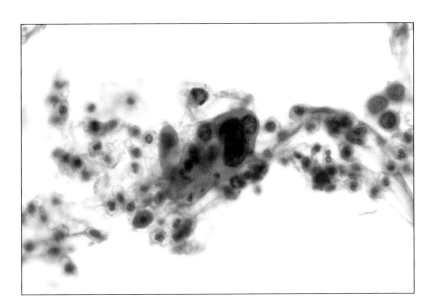

Figure 6.43

Squamous cell carcinoma

Pleomorphic keratinized and non-keratinized tumor cells are seen in a background of polymorphs and proteinaceous material (tumor diathesis). (Pap HP ThinPrep®)

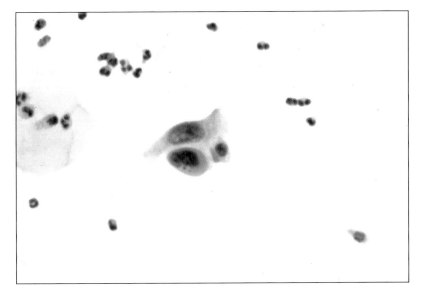

Figure 6.44

Squamous cell carcinoma

Three tumor cells are seen in this field. Indistinct nucleoli are present. (Pap HP SurePath®)

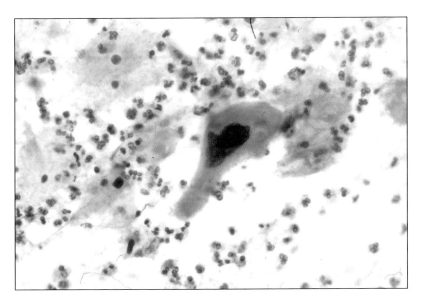

Figure 6.45

Squamous cell carcinoma

This is a large keratinizing squamous carcinoma cell with an irregular hyperchromatic nucleus, surrounded by tumor diathesis in the form of proteinaceous material, neutrophils, and cytoplasmic fragments, unlike the clumps of tumor diathesis seen in liquid-based preparations. (Pap HP Conventional smear)

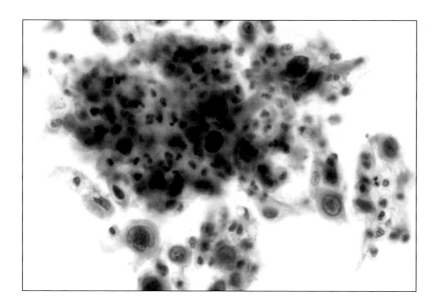

Figure 6.46

Tumor diathesis

A clump of degenerating keratinized tumor cells, polymorphs, and proteinaceous material constituting tumor diathesis, is surrounded by viable squamous carcinoma cells. (Pap HP ThinPrep®)

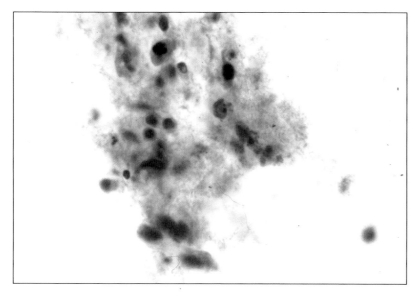

Figure 6.47

Tumor diathesis

Proteinaceous material and degenerated carcinoma cells comprising tumor diathesis are seen in a clump in ThinPrep® preparations. (Pap HP ThinPrep®)

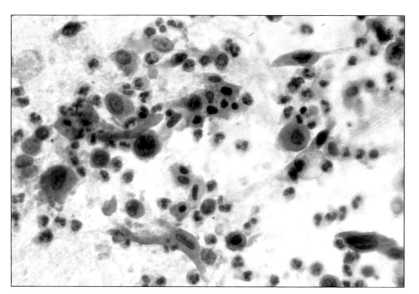

Figure 6.48

Tumor diathesis

Keratinized squamous carcinoma cells are seen in a 'dirty' background of tumor diathesis which consists of proteinaceous material, polymorphs, and blood. (Pap HP Conventional smear)

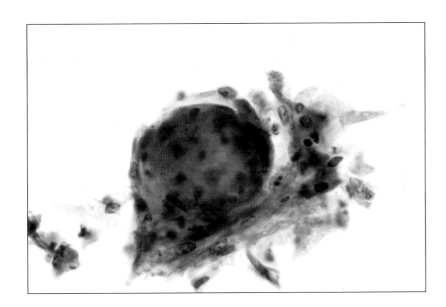

Figure 6.49

Squamous carcinoma pearl

In this field, a squamous epithelial pearl is surrounded by degenerating squamous carcinoma cells. (Pap HP ThinPrep®) Case courtesy of Charlotte Brahm, Cytyc Corp, Boxborough, MA.

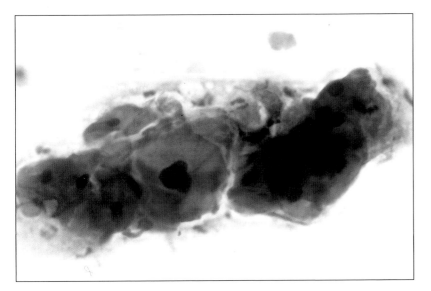

Figure 6.50

Vulval scrape, squamous cell carcinoma

These are keratinized cells that morphologically appear to be only mildly dysplastic. However, vulval smears usually contain cells that are of lower grade than the corresponding biopsy. (Pap HP Conventional smear)

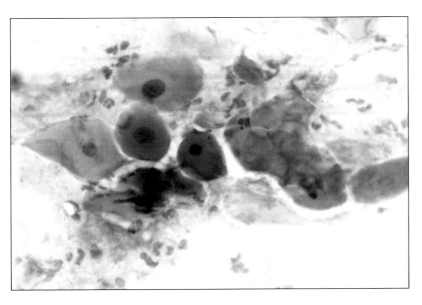

Figure 6.51

Vulval scrape, squamous cell carcinoma

This is another example of the LSIL appearance of squamous carcinoma in vulval scrapes. (Pap HP Conventional smear)

Recommended reading

1. Howell S, Theodor M, Pacey NF, et al. Quality assurance in cytology. Rescreening of previously negative smears from high grade squamous intraepithelial lesions. *Acta Cytol* 1997;**41**:1085–90.
2. Collins LC, Niloff J, Burke L, et al. Relative risk of high grade squamous intraepithelial lesion associated with prior abnormal Pap smears. *J Reprod Med* 2001;**46**:105–9.
3. Coker AL, Russell RB, Bond SM, et al. Adeno-associated virus is associated with a lower risk of high-grade cervical neoplasia. *Exp Mol Pathol* 2001;**70**:83–9.
4. Anderson MB, Jones BA. False positive cervicovaginal cytology. A follow-up study. *Acta Cytol* 1997;**41**:1697–700.
5. Mattosinho de Castro Ferraz M da G, Focchi J, Stavale JN, et al. Atypical glandular cells of undetermined significance. Cytologic predictive value for glandular involvement in high grade squamous intraepithelial lesions. *Acta Cytol* 2003;**47**:154–8.
6. Drijkoningen M, Meertens B, Lauweryns J. High grade squamous intraepithelial lesion (CIN3) with extension into the endocervical clefts. Difficulty of cytologic differentiation from adenocarcinoma *in situ*. *Acta Cytol* 1996;**40**:889–94.
7. Selvaggi SM. Cytologic features of high-grade squamous intraepithelial lesion involving endocervical glands on ThinPrep cytology. *Diagn Cytopathol* 2002;**26**:181–5.
8. August CZ, Ganji M, Froula E. Misdiagnosis of high-grade vulvar intraepithelial neoplasia (VIN III) as mild cervical intraepithelial neoplasia (CIN I) on Papanicolaou tests. *Arch Pathol Lab Med* 2003;**127**:68–70.
9. Clifford GM, Smith JS, Aguado T, Franceschi S. Comparison of HPV type distribution in high-grade cervical lesions and cervical cancer: a meta-analysis. *Br J Cancer* 2003;**89**:101–5.
10. Uyar DS, Eltabbakh GH, Mount SL. Positive predictive value of liquid-based and conventional cervical Papanicolaou smears reported as malignant. *Gynecol Oncol* 2003;**89**:227–32.
11. Singleton HM, Bell MC, Fremgen A, et al. Is there really a difference in survival of women with squamous cell carcinoma, adenocarcinoma and adenosquamous cell carcinoma of the cervix? *Cancer* 1995;**76**:1948–55.
12. Schreiner P, Siracky J. Estrogenic effect in vaginal sears in cancer of the uterine cervix. *Neoplasma* 1978;**25**:637–9.

7 Glandular cell abnormalities and other malignant lesions

According to the Bethesda 2001 classification, glandular cell abnormalities comprise the following categories: atypia, either not otherwise specified (NOS) (these are often just reactive changes) or favoring neoplastic; adenocarcinoma *in situ* (AIS); and invasive adenocarcinoma. (See Table 7.1.) There is no longer a category of atypical glandular cells of undetermined significance (AGUS).

Adenocarcinoma *in situ* (AIS)

AIS has typical features: increased numbers of hyperchromatic endocervical cell groups, crowding of nuclei, and fraying or feathering of the edges of the clusters. The nuclei are uniform in size and shape, vary from round to ovoid to elongated and contain speckled, granular, evenly dispersed chromatin. Mitoses are frequently observed. The cell clusters may show gland openings or may form rosettes. Strips of cells resembling the pseudostratification seen on biopsy may be present. Nucleoli are not a common feature.

Invasive adenocarcinoma

Features suggestive of invasive adenocarcinoma include three-dimensional clusters of cells with vacuolated cytoplasm and nuclei pushed to the periphery of the cluster. Nucleoli are often prominent and central, the nuclear chromatin varying

Table 7.1
Glandular cell abnormalities

Atypical glandular cells, not otherwise specified (NOS)
- Endocervical cells
- Endometrial cells
- Glandular cells

Atypical glandular cells, favoring neoplastic
- Endocervical cells
- Glandular cells

Endocervical adenocarcinoma *in situ* (AIS)

Adenocarcinoma
- Endocervical
- Endometrial
- Extrauterine
- NOS

from vesicular to granular. Tumor diathesis may be noted.

Endocervical adenocarcinomas tend to occur in younger women than do endometrial adenocarcinomas. They often have larger nuclei and may not be accompanied by blood and tumor diathesis. Endometrial carcinoma cells are smaller and are accompanied by histiocytes and blood, and, sometimes, benign-appearing endometrial cells. They more commonly contain phagocytosed neutrophil polymorphs. These tumors are more common in postmenopausal women. Metastatic adenocarcinoma to the cervix and vagina are not uncommon, the primary sites being ovary, breast, and colon.

Adenocarcinoma *in situ*

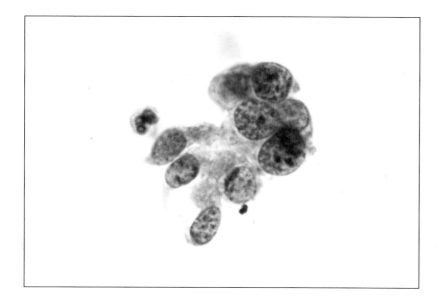

Figure 7.1

AIS

The cluster seen here is composed of cells with round nuclei, delicate cytoplasm, and clumped chromatin. The chromatin is typically granular in AIS. Note the polymorph as an indicator of nuclear size (normal endocervical cell nucleus is slightly larger than a polymorph) (Pap OI ThinPrep®)

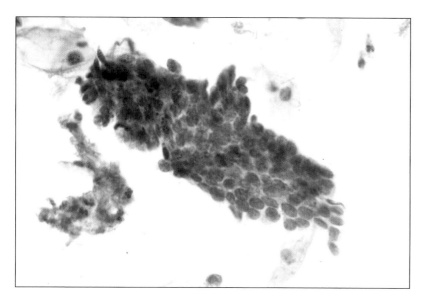

Figure 7.2

AIS

This tight cluster of endocervical cells shows crowding , overlapping, and hyperchromasia of the nuclei, as opposed to flat sheets with honeycombing and vesicular nuclei that are seen in normal endocervical cells. (Pap LP ThinPrep®)

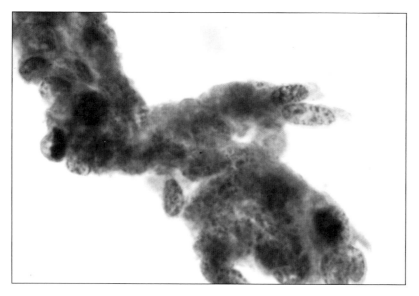

Figure 7.3

AIS

The neoplastic endocervical cells show crowding elongated nuclei with coarse, granular chromatin. No nucleoli are seen. (Pap OI ThinPrep®)

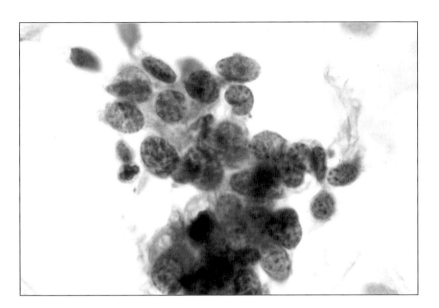

Figure 7.4

AIS

The endocervical nuclei in this image are also crowded with granular chromatin, but are more rounded in shape. (Pap OI ThinPrep®)

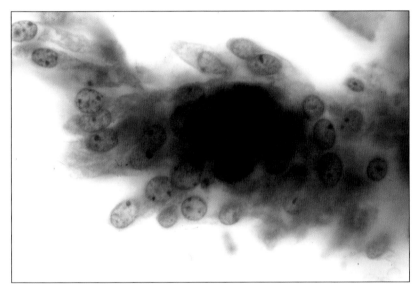

Figure 7.5

AIS

In this cluster, the endocervical cells at the edge give the appearance of fraying or feathering, a characteristic feature of AIS. (Pap HP ThinPrep®)

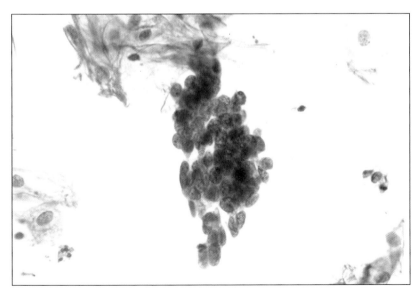

Figure 7.6

AIS

Crowding and hyperchromasia are evident even at low power. (Pap LP ThinPrep®)

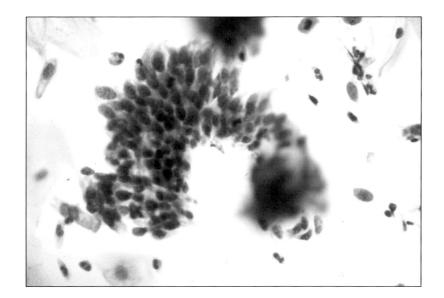

Figure 7.7

AIS

Crowded cluster of hyperchromatic endocervical cells showing fraying at the edges, in a SurePath® smear. (Pap LP SurePath®)

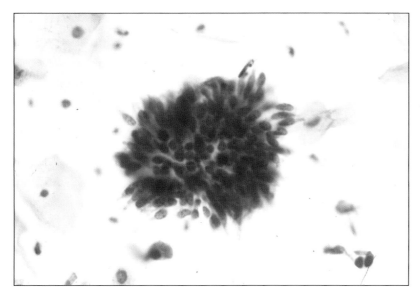

Figure 7.8

AIS

Another crowded cluster of endocervical cells with fraying/feathering of the edges in a SurePath® smear. (Pap LP SurePath®)

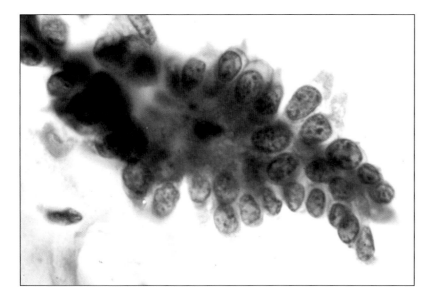

Figure 7.9

AIS

The cluster of neoplastic endocervical cells shown here exhibits ovoid nuclei and granular chromatin with fraying/feathering at the edges. Small nucleoli are present in some of the nuclei, a feature not typically seen in this lesion. (Pap HP ThinPrep®)

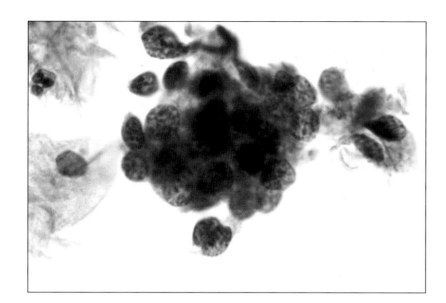

Figure 7.10

AIS

A three-dimensional cluster of endocervical cells showing the typical granular chromatin of AIS. (Pap HP ThinPrep®)

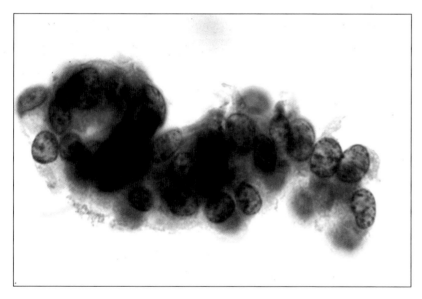

Figure 7.11

AIS

A strip of abnormal endocervical cells with a rosette at one end. The nuclei show granular chromatin. Rosettes are often seen in AIS, although in normal conventional smears they may be seen if an endocervical brush is used to obtain material. (Pap HP ThinPrep®)

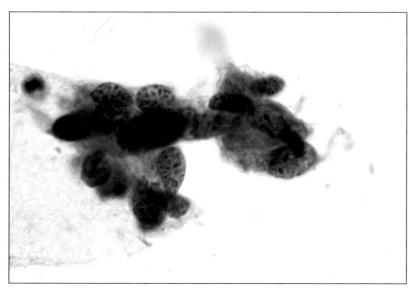

Figure 7.12

AIS

On the left of the cluster is a small rosette which is partially obscured by some overlying dark nuclei. Note the characteristic coarse chromatin of AIS cells. (Pap OI ThinPrep®)

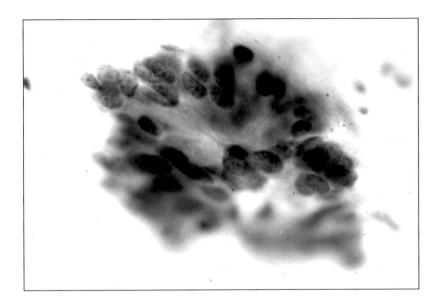

Figure 7.13

AIS

Conventional smear showing a rosette with elongated nuclei and stippled chromatin. (Pap HP Conventional smear)

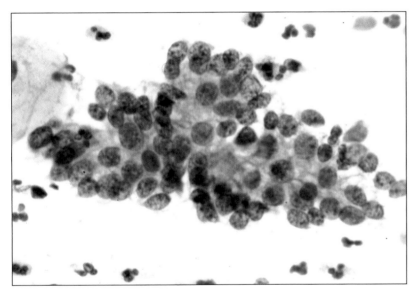

Figure 7.14

AIS

This loose cluster of abnormal cells gives the appearance of three or four small rosettes. The nuclei are small (slightly larger than the surrounding polymorphs) and display granular chromatin. (Pap HP Conventional smear)

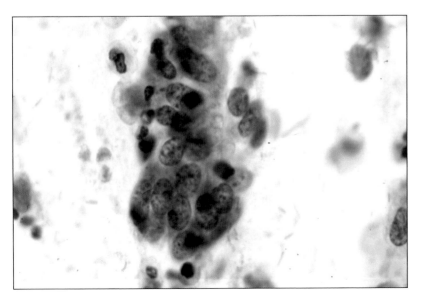

Figure 7.15

AIS

This appearance of layers of nuclei in a strip is the cytological equivalent of pseudostratification in biopsy specimens showing AIS. (Pap HP Conventional smear)

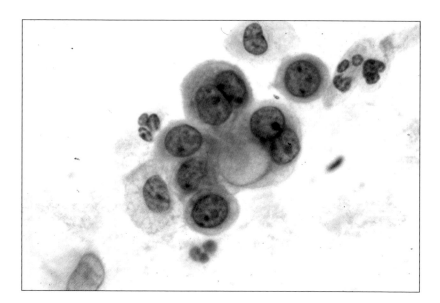

Figure 7.16

Endocervical adenocarcinoma

This cluster contains cells with round nuclear margins, somewhat clumped chromatin, nucleoli, and vacuoles. There is also some binucleation. Note that the nuclei are small, about the size of the adjacent polymorphs. Endocervical adenocarcinoma cells are, in general, larger that those of endometrial adenocarcinomas. (Pap HP ThinPrep®)

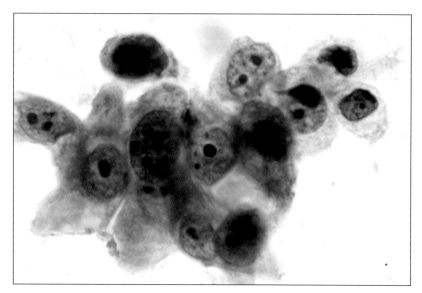

Figure 7.17

Endocervical adenocarcinoma

A sheet of neoplastic cells with enlarged but smooth nuclei, vesicular chromatin, and prominent central nucleoli. It is not possible to distinguish endocervical from endometrial or metastatic adenocarcinomas with certainty. (Pap HP ThinPrep®)

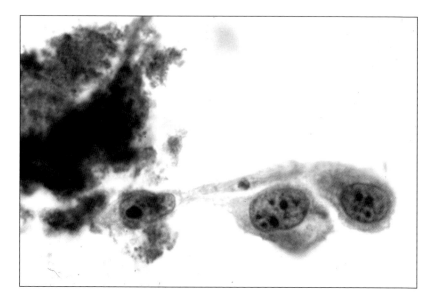

Figure 7.18

Endocervical adenocarcinoma

The three tumor cells show delicate cytoplasm and prominent nucleoli. Note the tumor diathesis on the left, composed of proteinaceous material and lysed red blood cells. (Pap HP ThinPrep®)

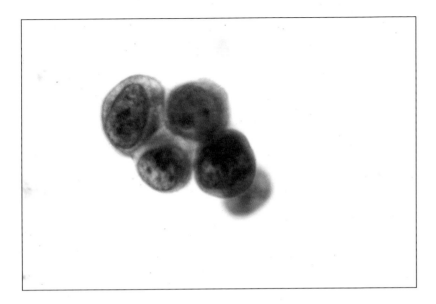

Figure 7.19

Endocervical adenocarcinoma

A small group of neoplastic cells with smooth nuclear outlines, clumped chromatin, and delicate cytoplasm. The differential diagnosis is adenocarcinoma versus severe dysplasia: these cells show small nucleoli favoring adenocarcinoma. Biopsy showed endocervical adenocarcinoma. (Pap HP ThinPrep®)

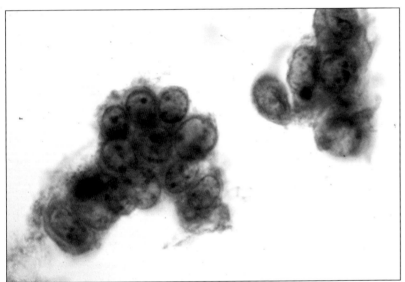

Figure 7.20

Endocervical adenocarcinoma

Clusters of glandular cells with nucleoli, pale chromatin, and wispy cytoplasm. (Pap OI ThinPrep®)

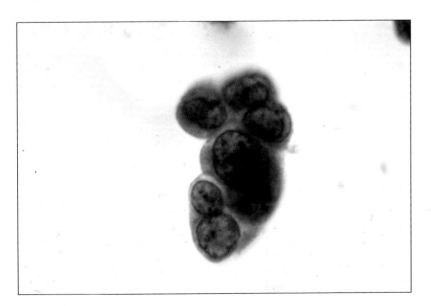

Figure 7.21

Endometrial adenocarcinoma

A cluster of cells is shown, with rounded nuclei and abnormal chromatin. The site of origin of the tumor cannot be determined from the morphology alone. (Pap OI ThinPrep®)

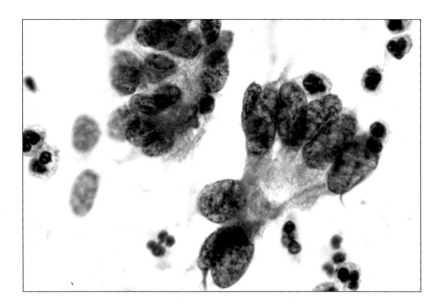

Figure 7.22

Endometrial adenocarcinoma

Two clusters of neoplastic glandular cells are seen forming imperfect acinar structures. The nuclei are larger than the adjacent polymorphs, are ovoid, and hyperchromatic. Nucleoli are not evident. These cells mimic AIS (Pap OI Conventional smear)

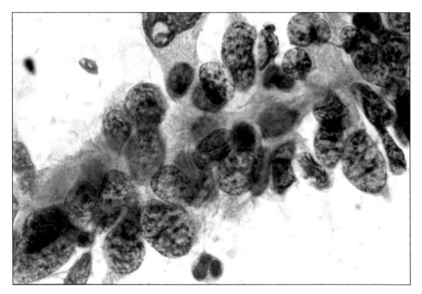

Figure 7.23

Endometrial adenocarcinoma

This elongated cluster is composed of cells with ovoid nuclei, clumped and cleared chromatin, and delicate cytoplasm. No nucleoli are seen. (Pap OI Conventional smear)

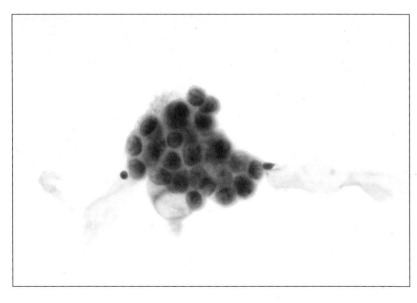

Figure 7.24

Endometrial adenocarcinoma

A cluster of glandular cells with overlapping nuclei and delicate cytoplasm; some nuclei contain nucleoli. Note the vacuole in one of the cells. These tumors generally have nuclei smaller than those of endocervical adenocarcinomas, and are often accompanied by benign-appearing endometrial cells and histiocytes. (Pap HP ThinPrep®)

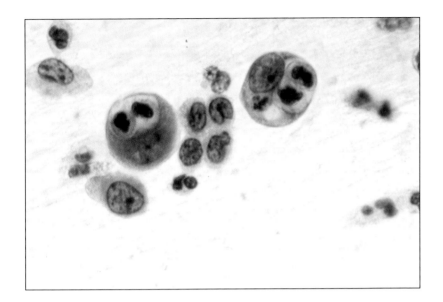

Figure 7.25

Endometrial adenocarcinoma

The two adenocarcinoma cells with eccentric nuclei display one of the typical features of adenocarcinoma: phagocytosed neutrophils. Note the small histiocytes that are the size of neutrophils in the field. (Pap OI Conventional smear)

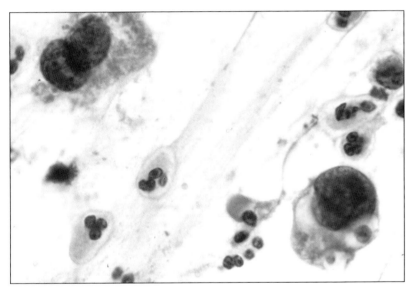

Figure 7.26

Endometrial adenocarcinoma, clear cell type

This conventional smear shows tumor cells with abundant clear-to-granular cytoplasm, accompanied by polymorphs. (Pap OI Conventional smear)

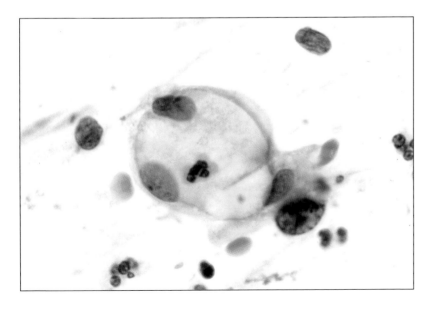

Figure 7.27

Endometrial adenocarcinoma, clear cell type

Same case as Figure 7.26. This field shows a cluster of tumor cells with clear cytoplasm and peripherally located nuclei that are not much larger than polymorphs. (Pap OI Conventional smear)

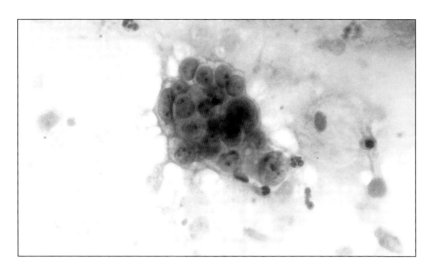

Figure 7.28

Metastatic ovarian carcinoma

This cluster of adenocarcinoma cells in a conventional smear was accompanied by psammoma bodies (Figure 7.29). (Pap HP Conventional smear)

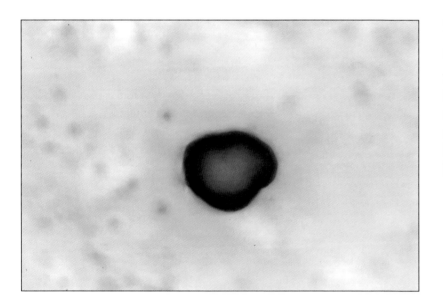

Figure 7.29

Psammoma body

The laminated psammoma body noted here was seen in the same conventional smear that contained adenocarcinoma cells (Figure 7.28). Note that psammoma bodies may be seen in negative smears. (Pap HP Conventional smear)

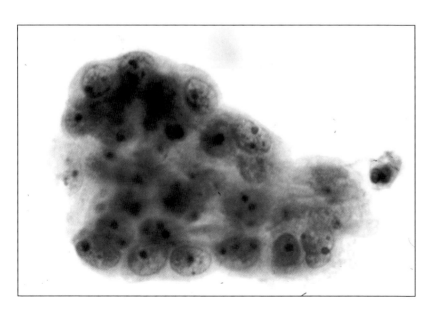

Figure 7.30

Metastatic ovarian carcinoma to vagina

This is a cluster of adenocarcinoma cells with prominent nucleoli. The primary site of the tumor cannot be identified by morphology alone. (Pap OI ThinPrep®)

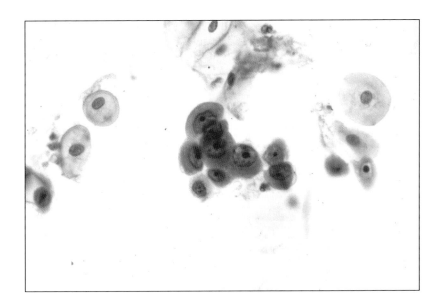

Figure 7.31

Metastatic ductal carcinoma to cervix

A cluster of adenocarcinoma cells with large nucleoli is seen in the center of the field, surrounded by parabasal cells. This smear is from a postmenopausal woman with biopsy-confirmed metastastic breast cancer to the cervix. (Pap HP ThinPrep®)

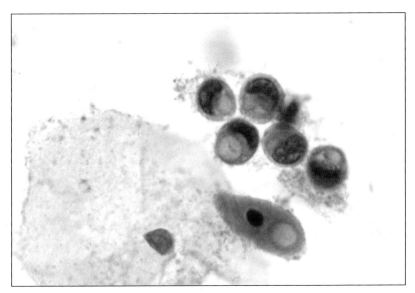

Figure 7.32

Metastatic lobular carcinoma to cervix

Five very small carcinoma cells are seen here, showing intracytoplasmic vacuoles and eccentric nuclei. Note the intermediate cell for size comparison. (Pap OI ThinPrep®)

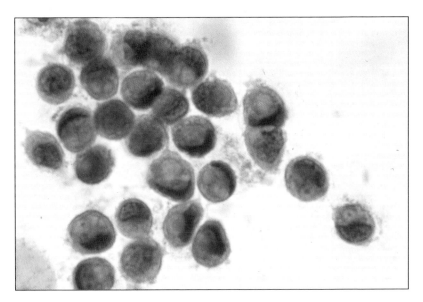

Figure 7.33

Metastatic lobular carcinoma to cervix

Several small lobular carcinoma cells with intracytoplasmic vacuoles, some showing a target-like appearance just as in primary lobular carcinoma of the breast. (Pap OI ThinPrep®)

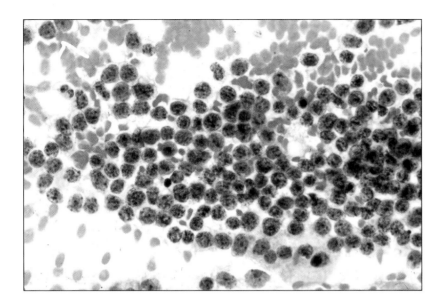

Figure 7.34

Lymphoma of the cervix

This conventional smear shows a monotonous population of small lymphoid cells, with no tingible body macrophages or histiocytes. Biopsy showed a B-cell lymphoma. (Pap HP Conventional smear)

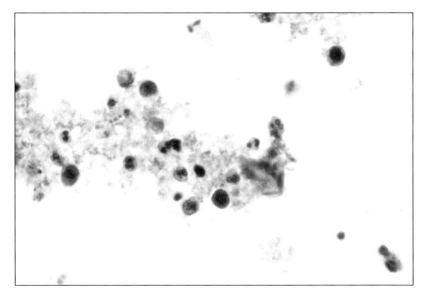

Figure 7.35

Lymphoma of the vagina

On low power, scattered lymphoid cells, neutrophils, and lysed blood are seen. (Pap LP ThinPrep®)

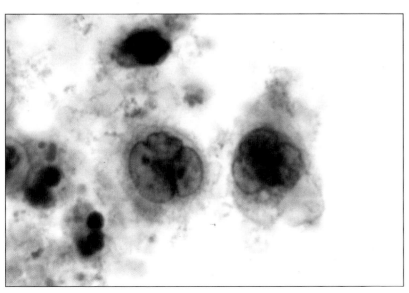

Figure 7.36

Lymphoma of the vagina

Large convoluted lymphoid cells with abnormal chromatin in a background of lysed blood. (Pap OI ThinPrep®)

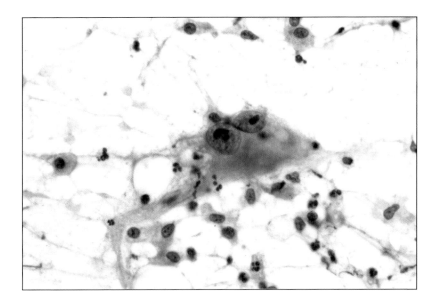

Figure 7.37

Leiomyosarcoma of the vulva

In the center of this field is a large abnormal binucleate cell with abundant cytoplasm and prominent nucleoli. Biopsy showed leiomyosarcoma of the vulva. (Pap HP Conventional smear)

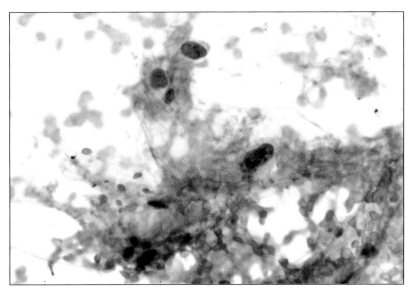

Figure 7.38

Mixed Müllerian tumor invading the cervix

Conventional smear containing scant tumor cells. In this field, the cells vary from spindle-shaped to more rounded with abundant cytoplasm. The biopsy diagnosis was mixed Müllerian tumor invading the cervix. (Pap HP Conventional smear)

Recommended reading

1. Burja IT, Thompson SK, Sawyer WL Jr, Shurbaji MS. Atypical glandular cells of undetermined significance on cervical smears. A study with cytohistologic correlation. *Acta Cytol* 1999;**43**:351–6.

2. Hecht JL, Sheets EE, Lee KR. Atypical glandular cells of undetermined significance in conventional cervical/vaginal smears and thin-layer preparations. *Cancer* 2002;**96**:1–4.

3. Krane JF, Lee KR, Sun D, et al. Atypical glandular cells of undetermined significance. Outcome predictions based on human papillomavirus testing. *Am J Clin Pathol* 2004;**121**:87–92.

4. Tam KR, Cheung AN, Liu KL, et al. A retrospective review on atypical glandular cells of undetermined significance (AGUS) using the Bethesda 2001 classification. *Gynecol Oncol* 2003;**91**:603–7.

5. Segal A, Frost FA, Miranda A, et al. Predictive value of diagnoses of endocervical glandular abnormalities in cervical smears. *Pathology* 2003;**35**:198–203.

6. Eltabbakh GH, Lipman JN, Mount SL, Morgan A. Significance of atypical glandular cells of undetermined significance on ThinPrep Papanicolaou smears. *Gynecol Oncol* 2000;**78**:245–50.

7. Levine L, Lucci JA 3rd, Dinh TV. Atypical glandular cells: new Bethesda Terminology and Management Guidelines. *Obstet Gynecol Surv* 2003;**58**:399–406.

8. Burja IT, Thompson SK, Sawyer WL Jr, Sjurbaji MS. Atypical glandular cells of undetermined significance on cervical smears. A study with cytohistologic correlation. *Acta Cytol* 1999;**43**:351–6.

9. Johnson TL, Kini SR. Endometrial metaplasia as a source of atypical glandular cells in cervicovaginal smears. *Diagn Cytopathol* 1996;**14**:25–31.

10. Chhieng DC, Elgert P, Cohen JM, Cangiarella JF. Clinical implications of atypical glandular cells of undetermined significance, favor endometrial origin. *Cancer* 2001;**93**:351–6.

11. Johnson JE, Rahemtulla A. Endocervical glandular neoplasia and its mimics in ThinPrep Pap tests. A descriptive study. *Acta Cytol* 1999;**43**:369–75.

12. Lee KR, Genest DR, Minter LJ, et al. Adenocarcinoma *in situ* in cervical smears with a small cell (endometrioid) pattern: distinction from cells directly sampled from the upper endocervical canal or lower segment of the endometrium. *Am J Clin Pathol* 1998;**111**:567–8.

13. Renshaw AA, Mody DR, Lozano RL, et al. Detection of adenocarcinoma *in situ* of the cervix in Papanicolaou tests: comparison of diagnostic accuracy with other high-grade lesions. *Arch Pathol Lab Med* 2004;**128**:153–7.

14. Schoolland M, Segal A, Allpress S, et al. Adenocarcinoma *in situ* of the cervix. *Cancer* 2002;**96**:330–7.

15. Riethdorf L, Riethdorf S, Lee KR, et al. Human papillomaviruses, expression of p16, and early endocervical glandular neoplasia. *Hum Pathol* 2002;**33**:899–904.

16. Hong SR, Park JS, Kim HS. Atypical glandular cells of undetermined significance in cervical smears after conization. Cytologic features differentiating them from adenocarcinoma *in situ*. *Acta Cytol* 2001;**45**:16–18.

17. DiTomasso JP, Ramzy I, Mody DR. Glandular lesions of the cervix. Validity of cytologic criteria used to differentiate reactive changes, glandular intraepithelial lesions and adenocarcinoma. *Acta Cytol* 1996;**40**:1127–35.

18. Schoolland M, Allpress S, Sterrett GF. Adenocarcinoma of the cervix. *Cancer* 2002;**25**:5–13.

19. Krane JF, Granter SR, Trask CE, et al. Papanicolaou smear sensitivity for the detection of adenocarcinoma of the cervix: a study of 49 cases. *Cancer* 2001;**93**:8–15.

20. Costa MJ, Kenny MB, Naib ZM. Cervicovaginal cytology in uterine adenocarcinoma and adenosquamous carcinoma. Comparison of cytologic and histologic findings. *Acta Cytol* 1991;**35**:127–34.

21. Erz W, Stoll P, Schrage R. Psammoma bodies in cytological vaginal smears in metastatic ovarian carcinoma. *Geburtshilfe Frauenheilkd* 1995;**55**:229–30.

22. Fujimoto I, Masubuchi S, Miwa H, et al. Psammoma bodies found in cervicovaginal and/or endometrial smears. *Acta Cytol* 1982;**26**:317–22.

23. Pauer HU, Viereck V, Burfeind P, et al. Uterine cervical metastasis of breast cancer: a rare complication that may be overlooked. *Onkologie* 2003;**26**:58–60.

24. Vadmal M, Brones C, Hajdu SL. Metastatic lobular carcinoma of the breast in a cervical-vaginal smear. *Acta Cytol* 1997;**41**:1236–7.

25. Taxy JB, Trujillo YP. Breast cancer metastatic to the uterus. Clinical manifestations of a rare event. *Arch Pathol Lab Med* 1994;**118**:819–21.

26. Mallow DW, Humphrey PA, Soper JT, Johnston WW. Metastatic lobular carcinoma of the breast diagnosed in cervicovaginal samples. A case report. *Acta Cytol* 1997;**41**:549–55.

27. Selvaggi LE, Di Vagno G, Loverro G, et al. Abnormal cervical PAP smear leading to the diagnosis of gastrointestinal cancer without cervico-vaginal metastases. *Eur J Gynaecol Oncol* 1993;**14**:398–401.

28. Casey MB, Caudill JL, Salamao DR. Cervicovaginal (Papanicolaou) smear findings in patients with malignant mixed Mullerian tumors. *Diagn Cytopathol* 2003;**28**:245–9.

29. Bokun R, Perkovic M, Bakotin J, et al. Cytology and histopathology of metastatic malignant melanoma involving a polyp on the uterine cervix. A case report. *Acta Cytol* 1985;**29**:612–15

30. Massoni EA, Hajdu SI. Cytology of primary and metastatic uterine sarcomas. *Acta Cytol* 1984;**28**:93–100.

Index

Numbers in italics refer to *tables* and *figures*.